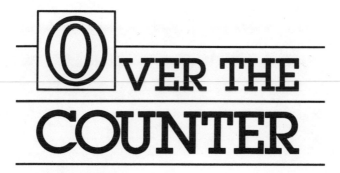

OVER THE COUNTER

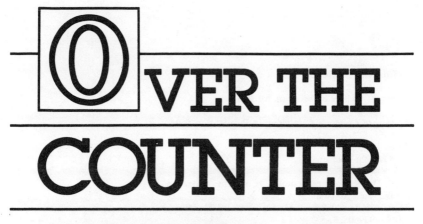

OVER THE COUNTER

*A pharmacist tells how to keep
your family healthy—and what
to do when it isn't*

DAN LITTLE
with Faye Lind

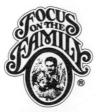

Publishing
Pomona, California

OVER THE COUNTER

Copyright © 1989 by Focus on the Family

Library of Congress Cataloging-in-Publication Data

Little, Dan, 1949—
  Over the counter.

  1. Drugs, Nonprescription. 2. Consumer education.
I. Lind, Fay. II. Title.
RM671.A1L58 1989   615.5'8   89-23751
ISBN 0-929608-30-5

Published by Focus on the Family Publishing, Pomona, CA 91799.

Distributed by Word, Inc., Dallas, Texas.

This book is not intended to replace a doctor's diagnosis. Any application of the recommendations made in the following pages is at the reader's discretion and sole risk.

Names and identifying factors about some of the people in this book have been changed to protect their privacy. The letters in Chapter 13 were edited for publication.

Designer: Timothy Jones

Printed in the United States of America

89 90 91 92 93 94 / 10 9 8 7 6 5 4 3 2 1

To my father, whose life and influence
were my example of my heavenly Father.

To my wife, who is my motivation and strength,
in this project, in my life,
and especially with our three children,
Danny, Christy, and Jennifer.

CONTENTS

ACKNOWLEDGMENTS

I'd like to thank the following people for their invaluable help. First, Ruth Rodgers, who transcribed the early stages of this book and gave me unfailing support and encouragement. Then, an enormous thanks to the editorial staff at Focus on the Family.

And, finally, a very special thanks to Dr. James Dobson for giving me the opportunity to share with readers over the counter.

LOST IN THE DRUGSTORE JUNGLE

I am at this moment
Deaf in the ears,
Hoarse in the throat,
Red in the nose,
Green in the gills,
Damp in the eyes,
Twitchy in the joints,
And fractious in temper
From a most intolerable
And oppressive cold.
—Author Unknown

"**I** am not going to go through another night like last night! If that man starts tossing and turning again, I'll hit him with the clock. He drove me crazy, and his coughing kept the kids up all night long!" Ada Adams muttered to herself as she stumbled out of her

1

car with bleary eyes and disheveled hair. It was a clear, crisp morning, and she felt eager to set things right. She strode into the drugstore determined to find relief for her husband's cold.

Wandering down the aisles, she scanned the brightly packaged products on the shelves. She felt as though she were wandering along the lanes at a carnival, with hawkers blaring at her from every direction. The products were all competing for her attention, all claiming to be the best. Her sense of confidence ebbed quickly.

Mrs. Adams glanced around for a helper. The clerk had her head down; she was busy with the money at the register. Behind the prescription counter, the phones were already ringing. The pharmacist was running his computer and starting the day's work.

They're busy. Let's see, what was that nighttime cough stuff I saw on TV? Oh yes, Vicks NyQuil. Here it is. And Contac 12 Hr. Capsules; that should help! Then I need some aspirin and vitamin C. I'll get the 1,000-milligram size. Here it is, with timed release. Great! With all this help, Walter should really be fixed up.

Mrs. Adams, with a little smile on her face, paid the clerk. She clutched her sack and sailed out the door, confident that she had achieved her goal. She was setting things right.

I have seen that scenario dozens of times every day in my thirteen years as a professional pharmacist. And I usually try to intervene before the purchases are made.

Let's review Mrs. Adams's innocent attempt to choose medications on her own. Her first mistake was thinking that because the pharmacist is busy she shouldn't bother him, especially if he is behind the counter. The rule is, "Bother him!" If he doesn't have time for you, get a new pharmacist.

Her second mistake was choosing over-the-counter medications on the basis of advertising. Hundreds of millions of dollars are spent every year on TV commercials that cunningly persuade viewers to try one product or another. The ads all sell hope. They are designed like ads for automobiles and underwear—strong on emotion and weak on facts.

Whether the medications work well or not, the ads certainly do. In 1982, almost $10 billion dollars of over-the-counter drugs and vitamins were purchased.[1]

If you buy a medication based on advertising, you may not cure the disease but create complications. For example, Vicks NyQuil is a "shotgun" medicine. It has four active ingredients aimed at every symptom associated with a cold. But if you don't have all the symptoms, you don't need all those ingredients. You are over-medicating yourself.

Worse yet, you are tippling and probably don't realize it. Vicks NyQuil is the only item besides bourbon that is fifty-proof, costs more than ten dollars a fifth, and is often taken straight in a shot glass. Check the label yourself; it is 25 percent alcohol. It should be sold in liquor stores along with Jack Daniels and Jim Beam! Instead, we sell it in pharmacies, to people of any age, without any warning.

I'm certainly not against the reasonable use of alcohol in medicine. However, one should be aware of the problems to guard against. Remember poor Mr. Adams, who is going to be dosed by his tender wife, whether he likes it or not. She is going to give him a shot of Vicks NyQuil with a timed-release Contac capsule.

If he looks at the capsule, he will see many little multicolored pellets. The pellets were designed with different thicknesses so they would dissolve at various rates and release the medicine over several hours. The alcohol in NyQuil, however, can strip all the pellets at once, releasing too much medicine too suddenly into poor Mr. Adams's system, and then leaving him with none for a long time. Moreover, when he takes Contac he should avoid alcoholic beverages, which means he shouldn't take Vicks NyQuil.

If you have only one body and you like it, you won't want to give it mixed drinks, such as alcohol, combined with medicine. I also warn people who take Antabuse (for alcoholism) about using Vicks NyQuil and other medications with alcohol content.

Many medications are affected by alcohol. I had a customer drink a beer with a 75 milligram, timed-release Indocin capsule, and within an hour he was very sick and nauseated.

"Of the 100 most frequently prescribed drugs," a 1979 FDA Drug Bulletin announced, "more than half contain at least one ingredient known to interact adversely with alcohol. Most adverse effects of alcohol-drug interactions are accidental, but the medical toll is high, including an estimated 2,500 deaths a year and 47,000 emergency room admissions a year."

Furthermore, if Mr. Adams is being treated for asthma, depression, diabetes, glaucoma, heart disease, high blood pressure or thyroid disease, or is having difficulty urinating due to an enlarged prostate, he shouldn't take Contac or Vicks NyQuil unless he checks with his doctor. The potential side effects or complications are too risky if he has any of the above mentioned medical problems or is taking certain prescribed drugs.[2]

At the same time, Mr. Adams shouldn't drive motor vehicles or operate machinery because these medicines will make him drowsy. And if he takes too much of either of these over-the-counter drugs, he might suffer dizziness, nervousness or sleeplessness.[3]

Surely the aspirin Mrs. Adams bought for her husband is pure and safe, you might think. But have you read the label on the pretty green NyQuil bottle? Even if you have, you may not be familiar with the word "acetaminophen." It's much like aspirin because it reduces fever and pain.

If you take Vicks NyQuil and aspirin at the same time, you are double-dosing. (No law exists against double-dosing, but most people don't knowingly choose to do it.) Further, if you intentionally double the recommended dose of both Vicks NyQuil and aspirin (which I certainly don't advise), you are really quadruple-dosing!

Of course some medicines can be readily mixed without a problem, but many times medicines intensify each other. Instead of getting an equation of $1 + 1 = 2$, you are getting $1 + 1 = 4$.

But the real point is that overmedicating isn't necessary. If you already take acetaminophen for pain and fever, you don't need to take aspirin for the same symptoms.

Surely Mrs. Adams was correct when she bought timed-release vitamin C, you may be thinking. So many kinds of vitamin C exist—ascorbic acid, sodium ascorbate, chewable, powdered, natural with rose hips.

Mrs. Adams chose the timed-release version because she had seen it advertised. Like most people, she didn't realize that absorption of vitamin C takes place mostly in the stomach. As the tablet glides gracefully through the intestinal tract releasing its vitamin C, the owner of the intestinal tract isn't absorbing much of the vitamin.

Even with the absorption issue cast aside, the question about the effectiveness of vitamin C helping with a cold has caused great debate in the medical world.

An old adage has it that people like Mr. Adams have two ways to get over a cold: "Properly treated, a cold will last about seven days. Neglected, it will hang on an entire week." I don't run into many people who neglect colds, so I don't know if that saying is true or not.

But I do know that cold treatment has made an entire industry healthy. Cold remedies are a billion-dollar-a-year business. The

Adamses of America have generously made that possible.

Mark Twain has given us an account of what it was like to medicate a cold a century ago, before we had our modern pharmaceutical industry:

> I went on borrowing handkerchiefs...and blowing them to atoms, as had been my custom in the early stages of my cold, until I came across a lady who had...from necessity acquired considerable skill in the treatment of simple "family complaints." I knew she must have had much experience, for she appeared to be a hundred and fifty years old.
>
> She mixed a concoction composed of molasses, aquafortis, turpentine, and various other drugs, and instructed me to take a wine-glass full of it every fifteen minutes. I never took but one dose...At the end of two days I was ready to go doctoring again. I took a few more unfailing remedies, and finally drove the cold from my head to my lungs.
>
> —Mark Twain, "Curing a Cold"[4]

I'd like to see what Mark Twain would say about cold medications today. Better yet, I'd like to see what he would say about medications in general.

With 80 to 90 percent of all health problems dealt with through the use of drugs, more than 1.5 billion new prescriptions are written annually, representing a sales volume of $17.3 billion in 1984.[5]

I call this a drug-happy culture, and I'm not talking about users of illegal drugs. I'm talking about normal, healthy, clean-living people like my own family, friends at work and folks at church. For example, here is an all-too-typical scene:

We start the morning with two cups of coffee to get us going. That's approximately 200 milligrams of caffeine. We then take our daily dose of self-medication at the breakfast table, from vitamin A to zinc.

Advertising has convinced women that they all need iron—and that only a maximum formula with twenty-six vitamins and minerals will keep them functioning to the end of the day. Next comes a diet aid that the mother takes openly, and a diet aid that her teenage daughter takes secretly. All this is ingested before 10 A.M. And by then it's time for a coffee break and more caffeine.

Oh, what a lunch! It is too good or too bad or too large or too quick, so out comes the Alka-Seltzer or Mylanta. In the mid-afternoon when it's time to meet with the boss or pick up the kids after school, it seems that a Valium or a Xanax will relieve the pressure.

In the evening we feel a little constipated (from all the iron we took at breakfast), so here come the Ex-Lax Pills or Doxidan. And at bedtime the sandman fails to show up, so Unisom Nighttime Sleep Aid sprinkles sleep-sand in our eyes.

I'm not exaggerating. When we Americans have any discomfort, we tend to *take something.* Our magazine ads, billboards, and television and radio commercials all tell us to live this way. No wonder our kids take drugs when they feel bored or hurt or uncomfortable. Their parents do—and often with the best intentions. Like my friend, Karen, whose husband, Steve, thought a certain medication would solve a little problem of his.

Steve's counselor had read glowing reports about a particular drug and thought it might perk up Steve, so the counselor asked the doctor to prescribe it. Steve figured it couldn't hurt to give it a try. But the drug didn't perk him up. It almost finished him off. Within twenty-four hours of starting the wonder drug, Steve noticed that everything was looking and feeling strange. After a sleepless night of near hysteria and odd sensations, he suddenly twisted into a kind of pretzel and groaned in agony.

Karen called the doctor who ordered a muscle relaxer for Steve. Karen rushed to her friendly neighborhood drugstore to pick up the prescription. She burst into the pharmacy with her face flushed and eyes flashing.

"I'll have your order ready in a minute," her pharmacist said.

"Please hurry," she begged. "Steve is having such terrible spasms I'm afraid he'll break his bones or choke to death!"

Off she ran with a couple of tablets in a bottle. In a half hour she returned to pay her druggist and to thank him for helping her. She radiated relief. Needless to say, Steve never wanted a refill for the "perk-up" prescription. He flushed the rest of it down the toilet.

Sometimes I agree with Dr. Oliver Wendell Holmes's famous claim that if all our medicines were dumped into the ocean, mankind would be better off and the fish would be worse off. But then I cast my eyes over the many bottles that mean life itself to some of my patrons.

As a result, I like and respect drugs because I like and respect people. Nonetheless, drugs are at once terrible and wonderful, like fire and ice. We appreciate fire, ice and drugs for the good they do, but we are wise to fear them as well. They can be dangerous, yet they sustain life, so we should respect them.

I realize that people have differing views about drugs and their usefulness. This is also true of a pharmacy. Some people think of a drugstore as a bright, clean, orderly laboratory. Others think of it as a novelty store with lots of interesting smells and sundries. And of course all of that is true. But I think of a pharmacy more as a stage where real comedy, drama and even tragedy take place week after week, year after year. It's a never-ending pageant of human life; and the pharmacist has a chance to be a friend, in a small way, to all the players.

I must admit, however, that my friendly pharmacy, like all pharmacies today, is also a chemical jungle. Every Steve and Mrs. Adams needs a guide in the jungle of drugs. I enjoy giving free advice and personal service to new drop-in customers and to my regular customers as well. I like leaning on the counter and chatting with them.

In this book I imagine myself leaning on the counter and chatting face to face with you. I want to help you cut through the overgrowth of products and advertising to find what you want and need. I want to clarify the confusion of technical terms and the tangle of professional jargon. I know that by the time you get to my pharmacy you may be confused, scared and really not feeling well. I plan to give you a personal view of what goes on and why.

I'll show you how to store your medication, and I'll even take you on an honest tour of my own family medicine cabinet. I'll discuss first-aid kits and safety caps and explain how prescriptions are written. I'll give you some of my own favorite health-care tips, and I'll tell you about some of my all-time favorite patrons and their poignant stories. I'll talk a bit about diet aids, vitamins, and pharmacy rules and rationale. I believe that almost any pharmacy customer is eager and able to understand more about what the professional health team wants to do for everyone.

There is no doubt about it: We are overmedicated and underinformed, yet today we have more health-care products, more advertising, and more regulations than ever before—and it's no wonder we have more confusion. So now let's enter the brightly lit, colorful aisles of your local pharmacy, and let me answer your questions so that you will feel confident about the many products on those shelves.

Worth Remembering

*A merry heart doeth good
like a medicine.*
—*Proverbs 17:22, KJV*

OVER-THE-COUNTER PRODUCTS: THREATS TO THE THROAT, SINUSES AND CHEST

After having spent a long day at work with a hacking cough that left him speechless, Mr. Parker stumbled into his local pharmacy, wandered down an aisle and began reading labels. "Ah," he sighed in relief, "this one alleviates coughing and pain of a sore throat. Just what I need!"

Then his eyes caught the words, "WARNING: May cause nervousness, dizziness, drowsiness or baldness. Do not take this product if you suffer from high blood pressure, kidney stones, swollen ankles or halitosis."

The words that followed were not much more comforting. "CAUTION: Avoid driving a motor vehicle, operating heavy machinery or using an electric can opener."

After a coughing spell that left him teary-eyed, Mr. Parker placed the remedy back on the shelf and began walking toward the door.

His pharmacist met him in the aisle with a friendly inquiry,

"Didn't you want that particular medicine today, Mr. Parker?"

Mr. Parker responded, "Are you kidding? Your medicine is hazardous to my health!" And with that, he stomped out of the store.

Sometimes an over-the-counter remedy fulfills the hope of the promised cure, sometimes it makes no difference, and sometimes it actually makes things worse. The difficulty, of course, is making the right selection from the plethora of choices.

Let's survey the possible medication choices—good, bad and indifferent—for Mr. Parker's sore throat. My father, who was a physician, swore by the old home-remedy of gargling with warm saltwater. It has worked for me for thirty-nine years.

When I suggest saltwater to customers, they usually look as if they don't believe me. It sounds too simple and too inexpensive to be true. But the saltwater is an "isotonic solution" in harmony with body fluids. It is soothing, helps the body fight infection and increases circulation in the throat.

I put about a half-teaspoon of salt in a cup of warm water (about eight ounces and as warm as you can use with comfort). Sip, gargle and spit out (don't swallow) the salty solution. Then rinse your mouth with clear water. Do this several times a day when you are fighting a sore throat.

When you feel like a gourmet gargle, combine saltwater with Chloraseptic Liquid (which comes in menthol or cherry flavors). Be sure to use water hot enough to heat the Chloraseptic Liquid. The result is a salty, cherry taste, but this gargle helps your throat.

It's too bad that little children can't gargle. Parents need to understand that and not try to force them. I have also found that children dislike most throat lozenges. I often advise mothers to give children a hard candy to suck on for a sore throat, because it keeps secretions flowing and the throat moist. Mild cough drops such as

Smith Brothers, Vicks and Children's Chloraseptic Lozenges are much like candy.

Actually, we have an odd custom in the United States of calling many of our throat lozenges "cough drops," when they do nothing at all for coughs. Their purpose is to soothe the throat. The one I use and recommend is Chloraseptic Lozenges. It comes in both menthol and cherry. Because it has phenol in it, it soothes the throat and helps the irritation.

Another good throat lozenge is Halls Mentho-Lyptus; it comes in five flavors: regular, cherry, honey-lemon, ice blue and spearmint. For choir singers, an old standby is Throat Discs. Even though they certainly work well, I can't stand the taste, which reminds me of a powerful licorice. They used to be called Parke-Davis Throat Discs, but Marion Laboratories produces them now. They are flat, pale and don't taste at all like candy.

Listerine Antiseptic Throat Lozenges, which come in regular or maximum strength, are another choice of many of my patrons. Best tasting, in my opinion, are the N'ice cough drops. They have a "slickery-smooth" taste, are available in several flavors, don't taste medicinal and are mildly soothing to the throat.

Mary Poppins sang, "A spoonful of sugar makes the medicine go down," but that's no help for diabetics and others who shouldn't have sugar.

Happy news for diabetics and dieters: sugar-free cough drops are now available. Cēpastat, N'ice and Halls Mentho-Lyptus are the most popular. Like most throat lozenges, they contain a variety of cooling agents or anesthetics, mild antiseptics and counter-irritant properties.

Some cough drops *do* aim at cough control. Of these, I recommend Hold, Robitussin-DM Cough Calmers, Vicks Cough Silencers and Sucrets Cough Control Formula. Another one I like is Mediquell Chewy Cough Squares, which are soft little squares with a cherry taste.

Most cough products contain dextromethorphan hydrobromide, often called "DM." It is a cough suppressant found in Robitussin-DM, Trind-DM and Novahistine DMX, which are all good. DM quiets the cough center, which is enough for mildly irritated bronchi.

One of the most famous and habit forming cough syrups is Terpin Hydrate Elixir, commonly called "G.I. gin." Many people receive relief after taking this product, even though it burns going down. I, however, would recommend this product only as a last resort because it contains 40 percent alcohol and brings with it all the liabilities of high alcoholic content.

If you have phlegm in your chest, you need an expectorant, which loosens and liquifies phlegm and helps the lungs expel it from the bronchial tree. The most common expectorant today is guaifenesin, in plain Robitussin syrup and in Congestac caplets. You should try not to suppress this kind of cough because it clears your lungs.

If you end up with a hacking cough that is dry, nagging or tiring, you probably need medication with something stronger in it, such as codeine. I think codeine is the best way to handle a cough, but the laws controlling it vary from state to state. In some states you can't get a drop of it in cough medicine without a prescription.

One of the most effective cough relievers available without a prescription is Benylin Cough Syrup, which contains diphen-hydramine hydrochloride. It used to be a prescription cough medicine. I recommend it to those who are so tired of coughing that they will tolerate the medicine's bad taste.

Few experiences can be more troubling than being awakened in the middle of the night by a child with a loud, barking cough.

I'll never forget the night my wife and I awoke in terror to the choking sound of our four-year-old son. The terrible sound came from deep in his chest. I can't adequately describe the sound, except that it was almost like an amplified bellow of a bull elk in the wilds. I panicked and called my dad, who was a doctor, to come to the rescue.

After asking me to repeat the symptoms, Dad asked me one question, "Do you have a humidifier?"

"A what?" I queried breathlessly.

"A humidifier," he replied calmly.

"I think we have one," I responded. "Why?"

"I want you to use it," he instructed. "His cough sounds so terrible because the upper airways of his lungs may be drying out. The dryness is causing the rattling that's such a frightening noise. The humidifier will moisten his upper airways and calm him down."

Desperate, I scrambled about for our humidifier. It seemed as if I couldn't get it going fast enough, but at last I had it set up by my son's bed. Within fifteen minutes, he was fast asleep, and we didn't hear another sound from him the rest of the night.

Since that time I've heard countless horror stories from other parents who have had similar experiences. Many of them have rushed their croupy children to the emergency room in the middle of the night and had antibiotics administered, which probably cost them between one hundred to one hundred-fifty dollars. In most cases, a humidifier would have alleviated the problem.

Now, I want to make it perfectly clear that using a humidifier is the place to start when a child has a croupy cough. My dad would have instructed me further if this simple procedure were not enough or if other signs were present.

I'm also talking about a humidifier, which provides natural moisture, as opposed to a vaporizer. A straight humidifier uses only water, whereas a vaporizer uses vapor medicine such as Vicks Vaposteam. Since children might play with a humidifier, it's much safer if the water contains no medicine. Otherwise, the solution could prove toxic to your children. In addition, a vaporizer is very hot, so it presents the danger of burning your child.

If you don't have a humidifier or a vaporizer, turning on your shower and bathroom faucets to produce a steam is the next best choice.

I have looked at ultrasonic humidifiers but have found that the only real difference between them and standard humidifiers is the water-particle size in the mist produced. Ultrasonic humidifiers put out smaller water particles, which benefit the patient because they reach farther into the irritated air passages.

The other improvements are mostly cosmetic and unnecessary, rather like extras on a new car. They include automatic humidity controls, easy to clean parts, musical night-lights and reusable air-filter systems. All these benefits double the cost of a standard humidifier; so you need to decide if you want these pluses bad enough to pay for them.

One practical tip when using a humidifier is to protect the table or chair you put it on with some kind of waterproof covering. Otherwise, you may end up with a soaked mess! I also suggest that you place a towel around the humidifier to absorb excess moisture.

If you are unaccustomed to the feeling of a humidifier in a room, you may be concerned that your child will contract pneumonia from all the dampness. You should have nothing to worry about, however, if you keep a light cover on your child.

Here are some words of caution regarding humidifiers: Your child may need more assistance than a simple humidifier can give, and a trip to the emergency room may be necessary. Use common sense in deciding whether you need medical intervention. If the humidifier doesn't make your child comfortable after a reasonable amount of time, please see a doctor, especially if the child has a fever.

Nose News

At least six hundred different cold viruses are known today, with new ones always coming along. A fair share of these affect not only the throat but also the sinuses.

Although I sell nose drops and sprays, I'm disturbed that most people overuse them. Overuse of these medications results in a condition known as "nasal rebound," which means the very symptoms you are fighting get worse.

Nose drops and sprays usually shrink and dry the nose lining. When a person uses too much of them, the lining sends a message to the brain, "Help! I'm getting too dry!" The body tries to lubricate the nose lining, which makes it swollen and wet again. The owner of the nose is apt to use even more drops or sprays at that point. This creates a vicious cycle which isn't very good for the nose or the purse.

My advice to patrons is that they not exceed the dosage recommended in the directions and that they not use nasal drops or spray more than a few days at a time. The spray I usually recommend is Afrin 12 Hour Nasal Spray, which should be used only as directed and for only a few days because it's strong.

The mildest nasal spray I know of is safe even for very young children. Called Ocean Mist, it's especially beneficial when a child's nose gets a bit dry, inflamed and crusty inside from low humidity. This spray is a mild saltwater solution that is soothing and healing, much like natural ocean spray.

Needless to say, the nose and sinus area is susceptible to colds.

Cold infections cause some of our cells to release histamine, which makes our noses swell and run and causes us to sneeze. The sinus cavities above and below the eyes accumulate fluid and start to hurt. Thus, we often take antihistamine to ease the symptoms.

A side effect of antihistamine is that it often makes us drowsy. That happens to me when I take my favorite cold remedy, Actifed. It's convenient because it comes in syrup, tablets and twelve-hour cold capsules. Other well-known antihistamines are Benadryl, Chlor-Trimeton and Dimetane, which give relief from allergies as well as colds.

When I was in the ninth grade, I was fortunate enough to attend the national Boy Scout Jamboree in Valley Forge, Pennsylvania. I had a wonderful time, but I broke out with a miserable red heat rash all over my legs because I had never been in such humidity before. I went to the medical tent for help, and the doctor gave me a small pink and white capsule. Now that I'm a pharmacist, I know that the capsule was Benadryl. I fell sound asleep for four hours, woke up confused and went back to sleep for another four hours— out cold. Even safe medications can pack a wallop for sensitive people.

Ironically, although decongestants can relieve cold symptoms, they tend to have the opposite side effect. Sudafed Plus can cause excitability in children and dizziness, nervousness or sleeplessness in adults. I heard from one young mother who couldn't sleep for three nights straight when she was taking Sudafed Plus.

Decongestants shrink the size of the mucous membrane that blocks the nasal airway. When sinus cavities become plugged, fluid backs up into the eustachian tube. The decongestant I like to use most is Ornex, which also contains some pain relief. I like it because it doesn't contain antihistamine, which makes me sleepy.

Once a patron, Mr. James, bought the strongest decongestant I had, with 120 milligrams of pseudoephedrine hydrochloride, to ease his sinus problem. Two days later he came back to see me, positioned himself close beside me and quietly confided that he couldn't urinate. This is a common side effect of very strong decongestants. I told him not to worry and suggested he stop taking his sinus medication. (Sometimes the cure is worse than the illness.)

Actually, most strong cold medications come in various strengths and formulas, and contain both an antihistamine and a decongestant. Actifed, Dimetapp, Drixoral and Dimetane Decongestant are some that I often recommend. Ryna Liquid is an excellent version for children over six years old who are sensitive to artificial coloring. (But be aware: Ryna-C and Ryna-CX contain artificial flavors and codeine phosphate, which may be habit forming.)

More and more products are labelled "dye free." In the past few years, patients, physicians and pharmacists have become increasingly aware that many people, particularly children, are sensitive to the different colored dyes that are used in many over-the-counter drugs, including some of the cough and cold preparations.

My main advice to you if you have a cold is to target your actual symptoms instead of using the shotgun approach. Don't settle for "one size fits all." List your symptoms, if necessary, and ask your pharmacist for help in finding the product that deals with how your cold is expressing itself. Let your pharmacist know if your sinuses are plugged, or if your ears are hurting, or if you have a cough, feel chest congestion or have a headache. The more specific you are in describing your symptoms, the more helpful the pharmacist can be.

If you are struggling with a runny nose, or watery eyes, or if you are experiencing a reaction to an insect bite or are displaying other hive-like symptoms, you want an antihistamine, such as Benadryl, Chlor-Trimeton or Dimetane. If you can't breathe through your nasal passages, develop pressure in the sinuses or experience fluid buildup in your ears, then you want a decongestant, such as Sudafed or Afrinol.

You will want acetaminophen—Tylenol, Extra-Strength Datril or Maximum Strength Panadol when you are feverish or develop aches from the cold. Panadol and Tylenol also offer a children's and junior strength for these symptoms.

If your cough is dry and hacking, use a cough-control product with dextromethorphan hydrobromide, such as Robitussin-DM. Benylin Cough Syrup and Benylin DM, with diphenhydramine hydrochloride, are also proper choices. If you are coughing up phlegm from the bronchial tubes, an expectorant is needed like Robitussin Guaifenesin Syrup.

Side effects may vary slightly from product to product, so be sure to check the label or ask your pharmacist or physician. It's also important to read the warnings for possible adverse physical reactions or for drug interaction precautions. Manufacturers are always bringing out new products or improved versions of the old ones, so check the labels regularly.

Pregnant or nursing mothers should be especially cautious and consult their doctors before taking all over-the-counter drugs, including cough, cold or decongestant products. (For more information on taking medications during pregnancy, see Chapter 13.)

Check the directions on medications for children; give them no more than the recommended dosage. Otherwise, they may experience adverse side effects. Follow age restrictions; some of these medications should not be given to children under the ages of six or twelve. And store all drugs out of the reach of children; a locked cabinet is the best.

The following chart will give you an overview of cough and cold products, when to use them and what their side effects might be. (The most recent edition of the *Physicians' Desk Reference for Nonprescription Drugs* was used to check information about the products listed in this chart as well as the remaining ones throughout this book.)

COUGH AND COLD

Product	When to Use	Side Effects and Warnings
Antihistamine only Benadryl* Dimetane* Chlor-Trimeton*	Hay fever, or upper respiratory allergy symptoms, rashes, insect bites, itchy or watery eyes, runny nose, sneezing or itching of the nose or throat	Drowsiness, dizziness, sleeplessness; check with a doctor before you use these products if you have asthma, glaucoma, emphysema, chronic pulmonary disease, shortness of breath, difficulty in breathing, heart disease, high blood pressure, thyroid disease or difficulty in urination due to an enlarged prostate.
Decongestant only Sudafed* Afrinol	Plugged sinuses or hay fever	See most of the above warnings; may cause racing of the heart, nervousness or excitability in kids; heart patients need to be careful; check with your doctor if you are taking medication for depression or high blood pressure before using these products.

*I use or recommend.

Product	When to Use	Side Effects and Warnings
Combination Actifed* Dimetapp Drixoral	All of the previously listed symptoms	See the previously listed side effects; watch for excitability in kids; avoid alcoholic beverages, driving motor vehicle or operating heavy machinery when using these products.
Decongestant with analgesic for headache Ornex* Sine-Aid Tylenol Sinus Medication	When headache or fever accompany cold	No antihistamine, therefore no drowsiness
Antihistamine, decongestant and analgesic Drixoral Plus Dimetapp Plus Caplets Comtrex	Need all three	See all of the previously listed side effects and warnings.
Cough control Delsym* Robitussin-DM* Mediquell Chewy Cough Squares	When cough is only concern	Check with your health care professional before taking these products if you have a cough due to smoking, asthma or emphysema or if you have excessive phlegm.
Cough control and expectorant Robittusin-DM* Cheracol D	Dry or hacking cough and phlegm present, no sinus involvement	See the previously listed warnings.
Expectorant and congestion Naldecon Ex Children's Syrup* Robitussin-PE Congestac*	Sinus congestion and phlegm present, need to cough to clear phlegm	See all of the previously listed side effects and warnings.

Product	When to Use	Side Effects and Warnings
Combination Robitussin-CF* Naldecon DX	Everything present	See all of the previously listed side effects and warnings.

Worth Remembering
Love and a cough cannot be hid.
—*George Herbert*[1]

MOUTH MATTERS AND SCALP SOLUTIONS

One day a woman came into my pharmacy toting a baby on her left hip. After searching our shelves to no avail, she approached the counter and inquired whether we carried Balmex Ointment for babies. I had never heard of Balmex, but after searching through my pharmaceutical catalogues, sure enough, I discovered the product was still on the market. I special-ordered a tube for the woman and didn't give the matter much thought. After all, baby ointment is baby ointment.

Two days after picking up the ointment, the woman came back into the pharmacy, raving about this wonderful product. I commented on how glad I was that it helped her baby's diaper rash.

"Oh," she said, laughing, "it wasn't for diaper rash; I used it to treat my cold sore."

That was how I discovered one of the most effective products for cold sores—Balmex Ointment. It also works wonders as a healing balm for minor burns, sunburns and chapped lips.

A desperate mother once visited my pharmacy with her little girl, who had a painful chapped ring around her mouth. They had tried everything from Blistex to Chap Stick without success. Knowing how Balmex had worked in treating cold sores, I suggested that the mother try it around her little girl's lips.

Within a few days the mother was back in my pharmacy, exclaiming about how wonderful Balmex is. The area around the girl's lips was almost completely healed.

Zilactin is another medication that works well in the treatment of chapped skin, cold sores and fever blisters.

For canker sore products, I recommend and use Kank-a. (I am not referring to a different product called Cankaid.) I can get rid of a canker sore in two days if I start using Kank-a as soon as the slight soreness begins.

To get the full effect of Kank-a, you must expose the sore on your lip and dry it off with a Q-tips cotton swab, holding the lip open and keeping the sore dry. Then you dab on a little Kank-a with the applicator from the bottle and let this coating dry for a moment. Doing all this at once is rather awkward, but it's a small price to pay for the wonderful relief that comes after several treatments. (If your sore is much developed before you begin the treatments, the Kank-a will be painful, and the healing will be slower.)

Proxigel and Gly-Oxide Liquid are also excellent products to use when suffering from canker sores. Another good product is Orabase with benzocaine. This is a paste that has the ability to adhere to the site of the sore.

Mouth Rinses

My dentist told me about a new toothpaste-mouth rinse. After I tried it, I liked it so well that I've been using it and recommending it ever since. Viadent (original formula without fluoride) controls dental plaque. The active ingredient is sanguinaria extract, an excellent product (dentists send in patients with prescriptions, even though Viadent doesn't require one). I also use the cinnamon flavor mouth rinse, which is very hot and refreshing.

Now, if I run out of Viadent toothpaste and have to go back to an ordinary brand, I find it too bland and foamy. For those who want a prescription product for bad plaque, a new one is called Peridex with chlorhexidine gluconate.

Another rinse I recommend is Phylorinal (one of the best, but it probably won't be out on the shelf—you'll need to ask for it or have it special-ordered).

The most popular mouthwash is Listerine. Named after Lord Lister, a great medical scientist, Listerine contains benzoic acid and 26.9 percent alcohol.

Oh, My Aching Tooth

For toothache, many of my customers have experienced relief with the use of ibuprofen (found in Advil). Most people find this analgesic to be more effective than aspirin. At least it takes the edge off the pain.

Another old-time remedy for toothache is a dental poultice. This little packet is soaked in water and then placed over the offending tooth. The moisture seeps down with the medicine into the cavity or broken tooth in a way that brings relief. Red Cross Toothache Medication provides relief when applied locally to the aching tooth with a cotton swab.

To prevent some of these painful toothaches, I heartily recommend dental floss to everyone. Most dentists recommend unwaxed floss, but most people buy waxed floss, which doesn't do the job as well. Special kinds of floss and instruments like floss threaders help people with bridges or other flossing problems. If teeth are tight, you need waxed floss because the unwaxed kind breaks and lodges between the teeth.

Other Mouth Sores

When patrons come in and ask me, "I have an awful sore under my dentures; what'll I do?" I have a good answer. I usually recommend a paste called Benzodent, which contains benzocaine. Several such products give patients relief. Orabase is another excellent product for gum and denture sores.

Occasionally people suffer from sores on their tongues. A gentle mouth cleanser and antiseptic sometimes provides the necessary healing properties. I often recommend Amosan as an effective rinse. Basically, Amosan is a hydrogen peroxide type of rinse that oxygenates the mouth and provides a chemical cleansing action. It is also good for canker sores, accidental injury or gum inflammation resulting from dental work. Verdesol is an excellent mouth rinse. All these products give your mouth a fresh feeling.

This Is the Way We Wash Our Hair

People and their hair vary tremendously. A shampoo that works great for one person is less satisfactory for another. The same conditioners that add body and bounce for some people seem to create oiliness or itching for the few who are extra sensitive.

I recommend that customers ignore the advertising and check out a few brands to locate one or two that give the best results. For sensitive people, simple shampoos, even baby shampoos, seem preferable. Some people claim their hair is healthier if they avoid hot water and hot air and keep their hair cool.

For those plagued with dandruff, the most effective treatment is the thick, black, sticky coal tar dissolved in shampoo. Yes, this is the same basic stuff used to repair and patch roofs. You can smell it a block away when it has been freshly used on a head or a roof. Today's coal tar or sulphur shampoos have fragrance added to try to mask the odor and conditioners to protect the hair from the harsh chemical. Despite the unpleasant smell, these products are still the best treatment for severe scalp conditions.

I would highly recommend that people thoroughly rinse their hair and scalp after using one of these tar or sulphur preparations. This will help prevent irritation and the smelly residue of these products.

Fortunately, a milder form of dandruff control works for most people—pyrithione zinc. The dandruff shampoo I use periodically is called Zincon. I alternate between that and regular shampoo. Pyrithione zinc is the active ingredient in Head & Shoulders Shampoo.

Sometimes customers want medicine to control a fungus infection of the scalp. A few doctors recommend the over-the-counter Tinactin Antifungal Solution for the scalp, but the directions on the box don't mention this use. If you are unlucky enough to have this problem (it could be called "athlete's scalp"), you'll probably want to ask a doctor to prescribe a strong antifungal medication to be taken orally or a solution to be applied topically to the scalp.

Bald, Balder, Balderdash

While baldness is not usually life threatening, men down through the centuries have been concerned about the amount of hair on their heads. Even the prophet Elisha in Old Testament times did not take kindly to being teased about his lack of hair, as evidenced by his calling on hungry bears to come to his rescue.

Two centuries ago, John Wesley, the founder of the Methodist church, sincerely prescribed daily applications of onion and honey to grow hair on a bald scalp. More recently, Tabasco sauce has been suggested for stimulating circulation and reviving hair follicles. So far all the home remedies have been disappointing, to say the least.

Turning to over-the-counter remedies, however, has not brought about the desired results either. Expensive baldness remedies are also sold to gullible people through mail-order companies or in certain barber shops, but no self-respecting pharmacist would stock them on the shelves. These remedies may promise to grow hair on a billiard ball, but they don't grow any really visible hair on a bald head.

Recently, a major development has occurred. Minoxidil, a new drug with the brand name of Loniten, was developed for high blood pressure. It had the surprising side effect, however, of growing a fuzzy type of hair on a number of individuals.

After many months of observation, a topical preparation and a powder made from crushed tablets of Loniten started appearing across the nation. Some preparations were chalky in appearance; others were of varying strengths because they were made in pharmacies and clinics in different ways. Nothing was standardized, and the company that had developed the drug was still holding the patent. After many threatened lawsuits and finally achievement of FDA approval, Upjohn released Rogaine as a topical solution for baldness.

But I do not recommend the use of Rogaine. First, this is a cosmetic preparation. Thinning hair or baldness is not a health problem. I have thinning hair and a bald spot on the back of my head. I am forty years old; it's okay for me to be bald!

Second, the medication is extremely expensive. The proper use of Rogaine can cost from fifty to a hundred dollars a month. The patient can't stop using it or the thinning and baldness returns. I personally don't have a thousand dollars a year to spend simply for hair-loss treatment.

Third, only a one-in-five chance exists that Rogaine will grow hair for a particular person. What does grow is usually a fuzzy crop of hair that creates a darkening effect.

Fourth, potential side effects include increased heart rate, aggravation of angina, excessive water and salt retention with weight gain and an irritated scalp. Furthermore, for those who take this drug orally, there is an 80 percent possibility of excessive hair growth on face, arms, back and legs after one or two months of continued use and close to a 100 percent possibility for those who take this drug for more than a year.[1] All in all, using this drug for baldness just doesn't add up for me.

Worth Remembering

Babies haven't any hair;
Old men's heads are just as bare;
Between the cradle and the grave
Lies a haircut and a shave.
—*Samuel Hoffersten* [2]

EYE AND EAR AIDS

Oh, the agony we put our eyes through. We stay out in the sun and wind too long. Or we strain our eyes in an endurance test by lots of swimming in a pool with chlorine in it. Worse yet, we spend a windy Saturday raking leaves in the yard, only to have a speck of something blow into the eye, where it then feels like a steel spike.

You've probably seen TV commercials for products that deal with these agonies by taking the red away. They are called "ocular decongestants." These products do their job by shrinking the red blood vessels to make the eyes appear white again, but they don't do much to help with the irritation. Repeated use of ocular decongestants can have a reverse effect, causing the blood vessels to open wider and thereby become redder.

I recommend an inexpensive eyewash named Collyrium for Fresh Eyes, which comes with an eye cup. The "miracle" ingredient is plain, cheap boric acid. In the old days, people had to boil, dilute and cool boric acid before using it as an eyewash. Collyrium for Fresh Eyes has done that preparation for you. It's good for eye irritation or tiredness, and it can be used to clear out little foreign objects such as an eyelash. This product is a mild wash that will soothe your eyes while you are waiting to see your physician for further treatment.

What can you do for your eyes if you can't use an eye cup or carry a six-ounce bottle of Collyrium for Fresh Eyes with you? I suggest Prefrin Liquifilm eye drops for tired, red, irritated eyes. It contains an ocular decongestant plus a mild anesthetic for comfort.

Another version of this product is Relief, which comes in a box of thirty one-dose containers. That makes it a convenient and sterile way to apply eye drops.

Few people are aware of two excellent eye ointments that can be bought without a prescription. The ointments are not usually out on display, but you can ask for them. Called Boric Acid 5% Ointment and yellow mercuric oxide 1 and 2%, they are good for crusty eyelids, irritated eyelids, sties and other minor eyelid infections. They can be used with children. Keep in mind, however, that they are no substitute for a visit to a physician and professional diagnosis.

"Artificial tears" are a true friend to unnaturally dry eyes. Some of the brand names are Tears Plus, Hypo Tears, Lacri-Lube S.O.P. and Tears Naturale II. These are all much like your normal eye fluid; they simply provide more of a good thing than your body is supplying for itself. You might have decreased eye fluid because of age, disease or a blocked tear duct. Artificial tears are an inexpensive, safe, easy way to increase eye comfort.

Here is another surprising fact about eye care: Most companies design their eye-drop products so that one drop is just the right amount for an eye. If you use two drops instead of one, the extra fluid triggers the tear response in your eye, and much of the medicine gets washed away. Yet some physicians direct people to use two or even three drops.

When I asked why, I was told that most patients miss the eye if they try to put in only one drop, especially if a parent is trying to put a drop into the eye of a squirming and blinking child. At least half the drop runs down the face, so doctors say two for good measure. If the drop goes in successfully, then one drop should be the ideal amount.

The Better to Hear You With

"My ear hurts, and I can't get to the doctor until Monday. What can you do to help me?" I always dread it when patrons come to me with that appeal because, to my knowledge, no over-the-counter product offers significant relief for ear pain caused by infection. I often have to say I can't offer any help at all.

I do have one piece of ear-advice to give. Several years ago, I got the first earache I have ever had. After an hour or two, I thought, "This is terrible. I need an antibiotic!" Since my dad was a doctor, I called him at his office and told him I needed an antibiotic right away for an ear infection. To my surprise, he didn't accept my self-diagnosis.

"Why don't you just take an Actifed?" he suggested. I wanted antibiotics, not Actifed, but since he was the doctor, I reluctantly obeyed. To my amazement, within an hour the ear felt fine. My eustachian tube (the little canal for draining fluid from the ear) had become plugged. The antihistamine and decongestant in Actifed opened the canal and removed the pressure that caused the pain. (Sudafed would have worked, too.)

The bad news is, this won't combat a real infection. My daughter came down with a mild fever and earache. One night, when it was too late to go to the doctor's office, her pain became severe. I was sure this did not warrant a trip to the emergency room and assumed I was right when Jennifer finally went to sleep after midnight.

The next day I took her to the pediatrician and learned Jennifer had a bad ear infection that punctured her eardrum before she went to sleep. The pediatrician was angry with me for not contacting her through her answering service in the middle of the night. I had been mistaken in assuming Jennifer's earache was nothing serious. As a result, I strongly recommend that you take no chances with ear infections.

Ear infections, however, are not the only reason for discomfort. Sometimes ear pain can merely be the result of ordinary buildup of ear wax. For some reason, people feel embarrassed as well as relieved to learn that their ear pain or diminished hearing is caused by ear wax.

A few years ago, as I was warming up my flash attachment to take a picture with my 35mm camera, I realized I was no longer hearing the little buzz that normally sounds during the warm-up process. After several months, the problem did not go away. I seemed to have lost the ability to hear high-pitched sounds out of my left ear.

Finally, I gained enough nerve to casually mention the problem to my dad. "Dad," I muttered, "I think I might have an ear problem. Do you think you could check it out for me?"

"Of course," he replied cheerfully. "Why don't you come on down to the office, and we'll have a look."

After taking a quick look in my ear, he confirmed his suspicion that I had a wax buildup and announced he was happy to clean it out for me.

I had been to my dad's office a thousand times before for various ailments and complaints. As he gathered the needed instruments for cleaning out my ear, however, I noticed they were unusually ominous looking. The tube he pulled out of his top drawer looked as though it were about twelve feet long. I shivered a little and then realized that it was actually only about a foot long and about an inch or two in diameter. A large rubber bulb was perched on the end of the tube. The instrument looked strangely like my mother's turkey baster.

I watched Dad as he slowly filled the tube with water. Then he asked me to lean over the sink while he positioned the tube at the opening of my ear. There was a sudden whoosh as he flushed the water into my ear. He insisted on repeating the process five or six more times. Just when I thought he might wash my brains out of my head, he proudly retrieved a chunk of earwax that measured about the size of a quarter. No wonder I couldn't hear my camera make music!

For several days my ear felt tender and irritated whenever it was exposed it to a direct draft or a mild breeze. Despite the discomfort, however, I was relieved to be hearing properly once again.

Over-the-counter products can assist you in removing earwax, but a doctor may be needed if the wax is especially stubborn. One of the most popular products is Debrox Drops, which is similar to hydrogen peroxide. It softens the wax, and then you flush it out gently with a syringe and warm water. Since few people have an ear syringe on hand, I recommend Murine Ear Wax Removal System because it comes with a syringe in the package.

Another ordinary ear problem is "swimmer's ear," a condition caused by excess wetness, hair sprays or an attempt to clean the ear canal. These conditions tend to disrupt the way the ear clears itself. Dirt and other particles collect and trap water, leading to an itchy, irritable condition. A couple of products, Auro-Dri and Swim-EAR, help dry excess water and help change the pH of the ear.

A physician should check the ear if you have pain or a discharge. He or she can properly clean the ear and treat it further, if necessary. This condition seems to crop up during the summer swimming season, so beware.

Worth Remembering

No eye has seen,
no ear has heard,
no mind has conceived
what God has prepared
for those who love him.
—1 Corinthians 2:9, NIV

CHAPTER

5

SKIN SAVERS
AND FOOT NOTES

They say that our skin is a separate organ of the body, like a heart or a kidney, but skin is stretched out all over us in a thin sheet. We tend to think of it as a Teflon shield, but in fact, many times the skin absorbs things right into our systems. You have taken drugs if you have rubbed ointment on your skin. Your skin influences your health, and your health influences your skin.

The Agony of Acne

One of the most frequent skin questions I receive is about acne treatment. For this skin problem, I advise you to use Aveeno Cleansing Bar for Acne or Neutrogena soap on the problem area when you go to bed at night. These soaps should be kept separate and used only as a medication for acne.

Another cleansing product that gives good results is Stri-Dex, which removes excess oil from the skin. Scrubs such as Brasivol and Oxy Clean are somewhat gritty and remove superficial skin but are also good. They work like fine scouring powder.

Next come drying agents such as Oxy-5 and Oxy-10. They contain benzoyl peroxide, which dries the acne. Start with the 5 percent solution, because this chemical is irritating, and your skin has to adjust to it before you use the 10 percent solution.

Dry and Clear is a well-known product of high quality. But OJ's Beauty Lotion is almost unheard of. I learned about it from a Christian psychologist who mentioned it on his radio program. It helped his skin when he was young, he said. I looked it up, saw it was still being made and ordered some for my store. Customers liked it.

Worried About Warts?

Warts are also a problem area. Many products advertised to remove warts contain acids, which can be harmful to normal skin. One product that has been around for years but still remains relatively effective is Compound W. Another product is Wart-Off. Since it provides a pin-point applicator and a little brush to apply the acid to the wart, it is more convenient.

Rashes and Chapped Skin

Whenever I talk about skin rash, an unforgettable encounter I had with a middle-aged lady, who spoke broken English, comes to mind. She seemed to think of me as a doctor in a clinic and always wanted me to diagnose and prescribe for her. I didn't mind giving her special attention until one particular day. She had a skin problem on her back and suddenly pulled off her dress so I could examine her back! They never warned us about *that* possibility in pharmacy school.

A little-known skin remedy some people swear by is a thick Vermont ointment used by owners of dairy cows. It comes in a bright green metal box with a picture of a cow and clover on the lid. The name is Bag Balm. It was made to be rubbed onto sore cow udders after milking, but people discovered that it was great for healing chapped or bruised human skin. Mildly antiseptic and soothing, it's even become popular at some ski resorts.

Your pharmacist can special order it for you if the drugstore doesn't carry it. The price is modest, and the container is an old-fashioned conversation piece.

Another good, old-fashioned aid is my standby, Balmex Ointment, which is great for diaper rash. Some mothers say it works better than anything else. (See Chapter 3 for a discussion of its other uses.)

Overexposed Skin

Quite a few people come to my pharmacy looking for sunburn relief. Products with aloe (from the aloe plant) are especially good for burns. It also helps if the aloe products have deadening agents in them to eliminate the pain, such as benzocaine or lidocaine. Check labels for the creams or gels that have a high percentage of aloe.

Sprays like Solarcaine or Americaine are also good pain relievers. But they are highly sensitizing, meaning they can make the skin even more sensitive by overuse. The key is to use them as directed and for a short period of time.

For direct contact burns from hot objects or flame, Foille ointment or spray is a good antiseptic and pain reliever. Neosporin topical ointment is also good. As the burn is healing, you should keep it clean and lightly covered for protection, with plenty of air getting to it.

An old home remedy for burns and bad skin bruises is ice water. It's amazing how much help this first-aid treatment can be. Put a pack filled with ice water on the skin as soon as you can. The cold water will constrict the blood vessels, ease the pain and reduce the swelling. Ice water in a pack also makes it possible to keep the burned spot cool while you are sleeping.

Another home remedy is putting butter on burned skin, but I hope this remedy is dying out. Most of our butter in the United States is salty, and salty oil is harmful to burned skin. The tradition must have started when butter was unsalted. Use cold water, not butter!

Aching Muscles

Analgesic creams and liniments are advertised and used for sore, aching muscles. You can probably recall those commercials that show an outline of a body with flames and arrows attacking the underlying muscles. These products, called counter-irritants, contain chemicals that irritate or "heat up," if you will, the topical nerve endings in the skin. The nerve endings send a message to the brain that the skin is irritated or "hot," which takes your mind off the underlying soreness of the muscles and gives a false relief. The muscles are still sore, but the nerve endings are more concerned with the heat on top of the skin.

Many people have used these sore muscle creams and liniments for years. I believe they can be effective with minor soreness and aching. Banalg and Myoflex Creme are two good products.

Of Soles and Toes

I have a friend who was studying abroad long ago and found

herself alone in Paris for a few days. She didn't know French, she had practically no money, and she suddenly got a bad case of athlete's foot that was raw, itchy and painful.

Without any real hope that it would help, she went into a Paris drugstore and started gesturing about her foot problem. The pharmacist and his clerks smiled confidently and presented her with an inexpensive tube of cream that worked like a miracle. Whatever the tube said in French, the cream looked and smelled like Tinactin Antifungal Cream.

My own daughter, Christy, got a mild case of athlete's foot not long ago, and I gave her a tube of Tinactin. She applied it regularly, and the problem cleared up in a week. Another excellent over-the-counter product for athlete's foot is Micatin, which comes in a cream, liquid spray and a powder deodorant spray. It used to require a prescription.

I average from three to ten athlete's-foot patients weekly. As somebody said, "There's lots of fungus among-us." Hot tennis shoes, colored socks and communal showers make the infection common among children and young adults.

White socks are the first line of defense because they absorb moisture and contain no dyes to irritate the skin. I recommend that children change socks when they get home from school and let their feet air out as they do so, whether or not athlete's foot is a problem.

If you contract athlete's foot, dry your feet carefully after your morning shower and apply a thin layer of Tinactin cream. (Putting more cream on does not make it work better.) Use this cream at least twice a day. Sprinkle some Tinactin powder in your socks as well as in your shoes if the problem is severe. Talcum powder will help to keep your skin dry, but medicated powder fights the fungus.

Be patient and faithful with this treatment. You may not see results right away; it can take two weeks to defeat the fungus. At first, the fungus might continue to get worse in spite of the treatment. If the fungus continues to get worse and worse, you should have a doctor check your foot because you might have a less common infection. Toenail or fingernail infections usually require internal antifungal medication from your physician.

Another foot problem that can cause significant discomfort is ingrown toenails. An ingrown toenail can be extremely painful for several days and occasionally may lead to infection. In rare cases, surgery may be required to relieve the situation.

I know of no medication that can actually remove the problem. Outgro is a helpful pain relief medication. It doesn't take away the ingrown toenail, but it does give some relief from the pain. If an ingrown nail is very sore and tender for several days, a visit to the physician is warranted. Soaking the toe in hot (not burning) water helps.

If you have diabetes or poor circulation, you need to be careful with ailments that have to do with warts, ingrown toenails or athlete's foot. A diabetic's circulation is compromised, so any of these mild conditions can lead to serious skin and circulatory problems. All these situations should be carefully monitored and observed by a physician.

Worth Remembering
You have made wide steps beneath my feet
so that I need never slip.
—Psalm 18:36, Living Bible

THE ABOMINABLE ABDOMEN

Stomachs are not as dignified as chests. In the dramatic opera *La Boheme,* beautiful Mimi coughed and wasted away in a Paris garret, and it made heartbreaking romance. But if her trouble had been in her digestive system, it might have wrecked the enchantment. Whether we are concerned with stomachaches or excess weight, we tend to feel a bit awkward about our abdomens. That's why we call them tummies.

Let's be frank about fat. It's similar to baldness in that people believe false promises regarding ways to get rid of it. I don't believe any good shortcuts to losing weight exist, including diet pills.

I get enraged when I see a television commercial with a slender woman, extolling the benefits of a certain brand of diet pills while claiming that her pharmacist recommended them. That's an insult to me and a disservice to my patrons. I sell diet pills reluctantly.

I had a plump customer who would come in to buy her diet pills while holding a bag of fresh doughnuts from the bakery down the street. I had another young lady who rushed in for diet pills every week, although she couldn't have weighed more than one hundred pounds.

Diet pills contain phenylpropanolamine hydrochloride, a decongestant that suppresses the appetite, but this drug should only be used for two weeks while you carefully cut down calorie intake with plans to keep the calories at a maintenance level after the diet.

Unusual reactions to phenylpropanolamine hydrochloride include nausea, vomiting, dizziness, headache, heart palpitations and tremors. It can also cause high blood pressure, restlessness and insomnia. Since this diet drug contains a decongestant, it has the same side effects. (See Chapter 2.) Warnings for pregnant or nursing mothers should also be checked. Common sense tells us that unnecessary medication is hard on the system and takes a toll of some kind sooner or later.

Now available are weight-loss aids like Fibre Trim that fills the stomach so that you feel less hunger. That is a vastly better choice, but it is expensive for what you get. You could just fill up on bulky natural foods like raw carrots or bran; however, if these products meet your needs better, I find no fault with them.

My advice to normal, healthy patients who want to lose weight is like a theme song: Buy a calorie-counter book and keep track of every bite you eat for one week. Find out how many calories you consume in an average day. If you are living on three thousand, plan to cut down to twenty-five hundred. If you are living on two thousand, cut down to seventeen hundred.

Don't plan to throw out all your favorite foods. Simply trim down your intake by avoiding temptation and developing your will power. This way you'll lose weight gradually and modify your appetite. This is being kind to your body.

Because I have been naturally thin most of my life, I have never needed to lose weight. In fact, I was too thin. I used the calorie-counting plan to put on weight, and it worked. I consciously trained myself to eat more than I felt I wanted. It seems to me that you can train yourself to eat less than you want in the same way.

Of course, some overweight people think it's not that simple. My wife, who has been overweight occasionally during her three pregnancies, insists that being too thin and having to force oneself to eat is a far different battle from denying oneself food when one is too fat. Even so, diet pills are not the answer.

Food is an emotional issue, and often a support group like Nutri-System, Tops (Take Off Pounds Safely) or Weight Watchers can be the most effective way to lose weight. Such programs help you know that others experience the same struggles and are in there rooting for you.

After the birth of our third child, my wife found she had gained sixty-two pounds. By faithfully remaining on the Weight Watchers program, she was able to drop down to one hundred ten pounds in about six months. The Weight Watchers program of providing recipes relies on a great deal of common sense.

Stomachaches

Antacids are another potentially harmful product. They aim to decrease or neutralize acid. Some contain aluminum hydroxide, which can cause constipation. Amphojel, ALternaGEL, and Basaljel fit into this category. No one wants to accumulate aluminum in the brain since it's possible that aluminum is associated with Alzheimer's disease.

Because some antacids contain magnesium, which can cause diarrhea, they also contain aluminum to counter the diarrhea. Gelusil, Maalox and Mylanta are this kind.

Some antacids contain calcium carbonate, which can cause constipation and rebound hyperacidity, which produces more stomach acid in the long run. Tums and Titralac are this type. Recently some physicians have been recommending these antacids as a source of calcium. These products do provide dietary calcium at a reasonable price, but users should be aware of the possible side effects. Long-term antacid use can harm diseased kidneys and change blood chemistry.

Antacids contain sodium, which many people need to avoid. Low-sodium or sodium-free antacids include Riopan Plus tablets or liquid, Tums and Tempo Soft Antacid. But they contain sugar. The best known sugar-free antacids are Titralac Antacid Tablets and Titralac Plus in liquid or tablets, which are also free of aluminum and sodium.

People ask me if one should use liquid or tablet antacids. The liquid tends to work faster and better, but the tablets are all right if they are chewed well and followed by a glass of water.

Antacids lower the acidity of the stomach and change its chemistry; they can cling to other medications. Patients, therefore, should check with their doctors and pharmacists about taking antacids along with other medications. For example, the antibiotic tetracycline doesn't get absorbed much if calcium and magnesium are present. Phenobarbital gets eliminated if you use bicarbonate of soda as your antacid.

Certain ailments call for temporary use of very strong antacids. The strongest ones are Gelusil-II, Mylanta-II and Maalox TC (therapeutic concentrate). Their use should be monitored by a physician.

Several antacid products have a plus added to the name. This usually means that they contain simethicone, a chemical that helps to break down and disperse painful gas bubbles. Simethicone is also available by itself in liquid or tablet form under the names Mylicon and Gas-X. Mylicon-80 is good for adults, while Mylicon drops or tablets (40-milligram strength) work well for adults or children. Some doctors prescribe Mylicon Drops for babies with colic.

ANTACIDS

Product	When to Use	Side Effects and Warnings
Aluminum Amphojel ALternaGEL	Heartburn, upset stomach or acid indigestion	Constipation; should not be taken with an antibiotic containing tetracycline
Magnesium Milk of Magnesia	Heartburn, acid indigestion, gastritis, hiatal hernia or peptic ulcer	Decreases effect of many prescription drugs; if you have colitis, chronic constipation, diarrhea, intestinal bleeding, symptoms of appendicitis or kidney disease, check with your doctor before taking this product.
Combination Riopan Plus* Mylanta* Tempo Soft Antacid	Low sodium diets best products to use; recommended for heartburn, hiatal hernia, gastritis or peptic ulcer	If you have kidney disease, check with a doctor first; do not take antacids when you are taking any form of tetracycline.
Calcium Carbonate Tums (sugar-free) Titralac	A source of calcium; taken for acid indigestion or sour or upset stomach	Constipation, rebound hyperacidity

*I use or recommend.

Product	When to Use	Side Effects and Warnings
Sodium Bicarbonate (Several brands)	Used for sour or upset stomach	Systemic effects (can be absorbed and affect blood chemistry); high sodium content
Strongest ANC (Acid Neutralizing Capacity) Mylanta-II Maalox TC Gelusil-II	Under medical supervision; acid indigestion or sour stomach with accompanying gas	Increased side effects; do not take if you have kidney disease or are taking any antibiotic with tetracycline

I imagine that when you wake up at night and realize that your intestinal track is playing a rugby match, you start to think about that pink stuff, advertised on TV, that comes cascading down into your stomach. Pepto-Bismol is popular, of course, but it contains an aspirin-like chemical that could cause trouble for ulcers if overused. Another standby is Kaopectate, which is good for minor diarrhea. It was recently reformulated; now its active ingredient is attapulgite instead of kaolin and pectin. Attapulgite has better absorbent qualities to stop the diarrhea and will also relieve stomach cramping.

Donnagel includes belladonna alkaloids, which also help to calm the cramping. But Donnagel can't be used by those with glaucoma. Parepectolin or Donnagel-PG are much stronger anti-diarrheal medicines that require a doctor's prescription in some states.

A new product has just been released that I would put at the front of the list for diarrhea. Imodium A-D is a liquid form of a prescription medication. It is strong; my patrons report it works very well. But any antidiarrheal medication is meant for brief use only, so a person with continuing diarrhea should see a physician.

While many people complain of diarrhea, many more complain of constipation. Laxatives are a multibillion-dollar industry, and Fleet disposable enemas are the single most frequently purchased item in drugstores!

I sell three kinds of laxatives. The first is the saline-type laxative, such as Milk of Magnesia, that causes water retention in the intestinal tract. Citrate of Magnesia, which comes in a ten-ounce bottle, is a beverage a bit like 7-Up and is to be drunk before colon exams. Saline-type laxatives like these can cause electrolyte imbalance, and I don't recommend them for general use.

The second type of laxative irritates or stimulates the bowels. It can be harsh, like old-fashioned cascara sagrada or castor oil. Milder types are Dulcolax and Doxidan. If you are recovering from surgery or are constipated by medication, I usually recommend either of those two. But if you buy Dulcolax suppositories, be forewarned that they work quickly, sometimes within fifteen minutes.

The third kind supplies bulk or substance to the intestinal tract, which pushes on the intestines' walls to stimulate peristalsis, the normal, wave-like motion of the intestinal tract. Bulk laxatives accomplish this naturally and help to establish or reestablish normal motion without chemical irritation.

The bulk-forming type is the best and the safest. Examples are Citrucel, Effer-Syllium and Metamucil. Even these should not be used long-term without your doctor's direction.

A stool softener is not a laxative, but it is needed at times, such as after a heart attack, surgery or childbirth. Most doctors recommend Colace, which is excellent. Because this has sodium in it, you must take that into account if you are supposed to avoid sodium.

I had a patient once whose son developed an inability to have a bowel movement without screaming and crying because his stools were so hard. He had been refusing to eliminate, and the longer this went on, the worse the problem became. The parents bought Colace liquid. Then, by bribing him with suckers, they convinced him to sit on the toilet long enough to accomplish the goal. The suckers provided the necessary incentive to work at regular movements, and within a couple of weeks, the problem was all over.

Many parents suffer needless anxiety about their children's bowel movements, especially when their children are infants. Some customers want mild laxatives for their babies. I had three children, and I never gave a baby a laxative. Under normal circumstances, it is best to give infants a chance to establish their own patterns.

Remember that diet, exercise and medications all affect elimination in people of any age. Don't be influenced by ads that try to make you think you have to use laxatives to look lively on the tennis court. Check your iron and medicine intake; they can cause constipation. Eat plenty of good roughage and fresh produce. Do lots of walking or other exercise.

LAXATIVES

Product	When to Use	Side Effects and Warnings
Bulk laxatives Metamucil* Effer-Syllium* Konsyl Citrucel	First laxative to use, safe, natural, bulk-forming	Should not use when you have abdominal pain, nausea or vomiting

Product	When to Use	Side Effects and Warnings
Irritant-Stimulant Doxidan* Dulcolax* Ex-Lax Pills	When a more moderate to severe medication is needed—in preparation for surgery or colon examination, after surgery, or for constipation due to other medication	Can cause dependency, perianal irritation, bloating, excessive bowel activity; do not use if abdominal pain, nausea or vomiting are present.
Saline Fleet Citrate of Magnesia	Only for an exam by a physician or under the direction of a physician	Do not take if you have appendicitis symptoms, inflamed bowel or intestinal blockage; check with doctor first if you have diabetes, heart disease, high blood pressure, colostomy or ileostomy, kidney disease, laxative habit or rectal bleeding.

*I recommend.

While we are discussing undignified topics, I want to mention the embarrassing subject of jock itch. I have had many an embarrassed patient lean across the counter and ask me in a whisper, "What can I do about this awful rash between my legs that is driving me crazy?" Jock itch is a fungal infection usually brought about by excess moisture, heat and lack of ventilation.

One day a relative called because he had a terrible case of jock itch. He was checking with me for assurance that his doctor was treating him correctly. This man is a teacher who has to spend his days in a hot room with no air-conditioning—a perfect environment for jock rash. His case was so bad that he had to be treated with internal, antifungal medicine as well as with external medication. If he had tackled the problem soon enough externally, he would not have had such a severe case.

My suggestions to take care of this problem early: Keep yourself extra clean and dry; change your underwear twice a day; apply a jock-itch cream after taking your morning shower and before going to bed. Use a jock-itch powder on your skin and in your underwear. Cruex, Micatin and Tinactin are the brands I recommend.

<u>**Worth Remembering**</u>

To eat is human; to digest, divine.
—*Charles Townsend Copeland* [1]

MAINTENANCE: VITAMINS AND MINERALS

One of the most frequent topics people ask pharmacists about is vitamins. People always want to know which supplements to take.

I'm fairly conservative when it comes to vitamins. It's my opinion that if you carefully plan balanced meals, adults and children alike are probably receiving all the vitamins and minerals necessary.

Obviously, if you suffer from a unique problem such as anemia or engage in detrimental behavior such as smoking, it will be important to supplement your diet with the necessary nutrients. Much of the advertising for vitamins found in popular prevention magazines, however, is often more hype than reality. In fact, ads such as those claiming that laetrile can cure cancer are downright dangerous, especially if they cause you to detour from traditional courses of treatment.

Whenever you see an ad or an article that claims certain vitamins or minerals have curative qualities, be sure to check it out before investing your life's fortune. Ask: Who wrote the article? What are that person's credentials? On what studies are these findings based? How long were those studies conducted? What is the scope of the studies? Through what products of nature are these vitamins and minerals available?

Most children, by eating vegetables and salads, will get enough nutrients to preclude taking large dosages of vitamins. The key to good health is balance, and if your meals consist of a balance of items from the major food groups, you shouldn't have to buy bottles and bottles of expensive supplements.

If you decide you want your family to take vitamins, my recommendations are as follows: For very young infants, I recommend Tri-Vi-Sol, which combines the three vitamins, A, D and C, that most babies need. Poly-Vi-Sol includes some B vitamins. If your baby is formula fed, check the ingredients in the formula. Often it contains all the vitamins necessary.

If you decide to give your children chewable vitamins, it doesn't really matter too much what brand you use. Sugar and dyes can cause some children problems, but for the most part there's little difference between Flintstones or Bugs Bunny—except the prices.

It's my opinion that the best nutrient supplements are the least expensive ones. All vitamin companies have to pass quality standards, so one is rarely that much better than the other. Most brand-name vitamins are no more beneficial than generic items. Also, synthetics are just as reliable as natural vitamins—and are less expensive.

Be careful not to overdose yourself. Taking vitamins every other day is usually sufficient. A higher vitamin intake can increase the possibility of allergic or sensitive reactions. I have seen rashes, welts and stomach problems result from too much vitamin intake.

You may be hypersensitive to a certain vitamin, like excess vitamin C. Or you may overdose yourself, especially with minerals like zinc or selenium. I also have seen patients react to certain companies' vitamins. Usually the problem stems from the manufacturing process, the inert ingredients (the nonactive parts of a tablet) or even the coloring used in the products.

I recommend vitamins for limited, specific use only and not for prevention of possible diseases. Some people swear that large dosages of vitamin C help to prevent a cold. I don't think anyone should take more than 500 milligrams at a time. We do know that vitamin C can aggravate an ulcer condition and can change the chemistry of the urine, affecting the kidney's ability to eliminate certain medications. Be careful with the amount you take.

Another area of concern, especially for women, is calcium intake and the prevention of osteoporosis. I think that if women drink at least a glass of milk a day, they won't need calcium supplements.

But if you decide you'd rather get your calcium through a supplement, several options are available: Os-Cal, a natural source of calcium carbonate; Posture Calcium, which eliminates stomach upset; Calcet, which combines three kinds of calcium into one tablet; and Calcet Plus, which adds vitamins along with the calcium. Many doctors are suggesting people take antacids like Titralac or Tums for their calcium intake, but there are potential negative side effects. (See Chapter 6.)

A recent study evaluated the effectiveness of various brands of calcium supplements. Dr. Ralph F. Shangraw, the chairman of the department of pharmaceutics at the University of Maryland School of Pharmacy, has released some eye-opening results of experiments to find out if calcium supplements dissolve in time to be absorbed.

Calcium tablets need to be 75 percent dissolved within thirty minutes or they will be ineffective. But many of the brands tested were way below the 75 percent level, with some as low as 2 percent dissolved. In other words, those calcium tablets provided no benefit to the taker.

Some of the more promising brands, with 100 percent dissolution in thirty minutes, were Marion Laboratories' Os-Cal and Norcliff Thayer's Tums.

Several of the companies that received poor marks on their calcium products have reformulated their tablets, so we should be receiving better products as a result of these experiments.

A simple test for your favorite calcium product is to take one of your tablets and place it in white distilled vinegar for thirty minutes. If it doesn't completely dissolve, you probably should change products.

One other calcium product you might buy is Calcilyte, an effervescent tablet that is dissolved in water before you take it. This product is a little more expensive, but it is worth it. It uses calcium citrate as its calcium source. Even though calcium carbonate is one of the most concentrated sources of calcium, calcium citrate is one of the best absorbed.

Whatever form of calcium you decide to take, do so with a good meal or a glass of water or juice. This helps dissolve the tablets more efficiently.

My main recommendation regarding vitamins and mineral supplements is to get your nutrients from natural sources, the food you eat, rather than from pills. If you must take supplements, buy from the most economical source you can. Don't go with every fad; use common sense.

Following is a chart to help summarize my recommendations for children and adults, if you decide to use vitamins:

VITAMINS

Product	Contains	Special Notes
For infants:		Iron should be given
Tri-Vi-Sol	A, D, C	only if baby is anemic
Poly-Vi-Sol	A, D, C, E, B6, B12 and Niacin	or if recommended by doctor
Cecon	C	
Ce-Vi-Sol	C	
For children:		
Chewable multi-vitamins		
Bugs Bunny (sugar free)		
Flintstones		
Poly-Vi-Sol		
Theragran Jr. (sugar free)		
Vi-Daylin		
Store brand		
Chewable vitamin C		Give young children no more than 100 milligrams; older children and teens no more than 250 milligrams; maximum amount with a cold 500 milligrams
Liquid vitamins		
Vi-Daylin Drops		
Vi-Daylin ADC Drops		
Calcium		
Neo-Calglucon		A liquid source of calcium for children who are allergic to dairy products
For adults:		
Multi-vitamins		
Myadec		
Theragran-M		
Unicap		
Store brands		

Product	Contains	Special Notes
Calcium		
Posture Calcium		Designed for sensitive stomachs
Calcet	Source of calcium, but also helps leg cramps	
Os-Cal		
Store brands		
Oyster shell brands		Favorite of many doctors
Titralac	Antacid used as source of calcium	Long-term use can harm diseased kidneys and change blood chemistry
Tums	Antacid used as source of calcium	Long-term use can harm diseased kidneys and change blood chemistry
Vitamin C		Take no more than 500 milligrams; 1,000 milligrams maximum with a cold

Cholesterol Concerns

In addition to the vitamin craze, more and more people are concerned about cholesterol—it's the new rage. Now, I'm all for lowering the cholesterol in your diet. I encourage you to change to low-fat or nonfat milk and to eat less ice cream.

The first thing you should do, however, is go to a physician and get a blood test that specifically shows your cholesterol levels. Once you discover your cholesterol level, ask your doctor whether he or she would consider it within the normal range. Doctors differ greatly as to what they consider normal cholesterol levels.

These levels are measured as so many milligrams per 100 milliliters of serum. A level of 150 milligrams per 100 milliliters to 250 milligrams per 100 milliliters of cholesterol is considered normal. Thus 200 milligrams per 100 milliliters is middle ground. But depending on age, existing medical conditions and familial history, this level may still be too high.

If you discover your level is about 220, then I would suggest you start watching your diet carefully. After checking with your doctor, you might try fish-oil capsules or increase your intake of oat bran. Then go back to your doctor in three months to have your cholesterol level tested once again. If your level has lowered, then continue your diet and fish-oil capsules.

Fluoride Facts

It's important that your child receive the correct amount of fluoride. If too much fluoride is given, it can eventually discolor your child's teeth; if too little is given, your child will be more susceptible to cavities.

To strike a balance, find out the fluoride content in your local water supply. Simply call your local water department. Then check with your pediatric dentist for his or her recommendations as to how much fluoride is necessary. If you discover the fluoride content is low, have your doctor prescribe the necessary amount.

We have looked at remedies for all kinds of ailments. But whatever the ailments are, most are apt to cause some pain. As a wise person observed, the only trouble with pain is that it hurts. In the next chapter we will look more closely at ways to relieve pain.

Worth Remembering
Look to your health; and if you have it,
praise God, and value it next to a good conscience.
—*Izaak Walton*[1]

CAN YOU TAKE AWAY THE PAIN?

Sooner or later, we all want relief from big or little pains. The medications we can choose from run the gamut—from A to Z, from aspirin to Zomax. But most people end up back at aspirin most of the time.

In the early 1980s, Zomax was advertised as the "after-aspirin" painkiller—newer, much stronger and nonaddictive. But Zomax was taken off the market after fifteen million patients had used it, because some people went into shock and a few died. That new answer to pain faded fast, but researchers are constantly working to develop new, improved analgesics that will prove more valuable.

I suspect that some people wonder what the word "analgesic" really means but feel embarrassed to ask. "Analgesic" is not a modern scientific concept; it's just Greek for "pain remover." Druggists tend to call themselves "pharmacists" and call painkillers "analgesics." But "druggist" and "painkiller" are just as correct. Whether people know the word "analgesic" or not, everyone knows the name of our favorite analgesic, aspirin.

The search for such a painkiller began centuries before aspirin was discovered. Hippocrates, the father of modern medicine, found that willow leaves relieved pain, and he recommended that women chew on them during childbirth. We now know that willow leaves contain salicin, a property of aspirin. Then, in 1757, Reverend Edmund Stone experimented with willow bark and found that it brought down malarial fevers. His discovery, which was reported in a London journal, was one of the first modern steps toward the development of aspirin.

By 1874, salicylic acid, a crude drug, was being used to relieve pain and lower fevers. But it also burned the mouth and throat and caused severe nausea. Almost twenty years later, Felix Hoffman, a German research chemist, was asked by his company to find a painkiller that didn't have such irritating side effects. He had a personal motivation to discover a painkiller as well. His father, who had rheumatoid arthritis, couldn't tolerate salicylate because of its adverse side effects.

Hoffman developed and then tested acetylsalicylic acid on himself and his father and found that it relieved pain without burning the mouth or causing nausea. So in 1899, the new drug was launched, but because acetylsalicylic acid was too difficult to pronounce or remember, Hoffman and his colleagues named the product "aspirin."[1]

Also at the turn of the century, Freud's psychoanalytic theories hit the press and started to sweep the world. Things haven't been the same since. Some people think we got our worst headache and our best headache medicine at the same time.

Until recently, aspirin was by far the most commonly used, effective painkiller one could buy without a prescription. It was such a universal answer to pain and fever that few people realized it did not work for everyone.

An unknown percentage of people get no relief at all from aspirin, and two out of a thousand people are dangerously allergic to it, especially those who have asthma or suffer from hives. (Some allergists think aspirin should be a prescription drug.) For people in this group, "Take two aspirin tablets and call me in the morning" is a sad joke.

Four more groups should also do without aspirin. First, children who have an acute case of viral infection such as the flu, chicken pox or upper respiratory infection should not receive aspirin because of a possible link between these illnesses, aspirin and Reye's syndrome.

Symptoms of Reye's syndrome come in progressive stages and appear within one to three days following one of the above infections. After the child seems to have recovered from the infection, he or she will develop persistent vomiting, agitation, belligerence, hyperactivity, mental confusion and, finally, coma.[2] The death rate is about 30 percent, and survivors are apt to have permanent brain damage. Even though Reye's syndrome is rare, parents should be cautious about giving aspirin to their sick children and teenagers until more is known about this problem.

One night recently my daughter, Christy, woke up with a temperature of 104 degrees. I was in a rush to lower that fever. In the past I would have given her aspirin because it's fast and effective for high fevers, but this time I gave her the slower Tylenol (acetaminophen) instead. I didn't know what she was fighting, and I didn't want to risk Reye's syndrome.

The second group which should be careful about the use of aspirin are those who have gout. If you have this condition, you should be aware that low doses of aspirin can make your problem worse instead of better. Third, if you take medications, you should check with your physician to make sure that aspirin won't conflict with your other medicine.

Four, if you have stomach trouble, you need to watch your aspirin intake. Some experts think that every time you take an aspirin you cause a little bleeding in your stomach. This could be dangerous if you have a tendency toward ulcers.

If you need to protect your stomach, I recommend special aspirins like Ascriptin and Bufferin because they contain antacid. Some aspirins like Ecotrin have a heavy coating that keeps the aspirin from contacting the stomach and delays its absorption until it goes farther down the digestive tract. This is good if you have to take large quantities of aspirin. But beware, they can cause intestinal ulcers.

A final warning regarding aspirin: An overdose can poison or even cause death in children or adults. Using bottles with childproof safety caps and storing aspirin in a locked cabinet will help to reduce the incidence of accidental poisoning in children.

The analgesic acetaminophen is much safer, and it doesn't irritate the stomach. Acetaminophen, the prime substitute for aspirin, is the analgesic in Tylenol, Panadol, Tempra and Datril. For most purposes, acetaminophen is a good substitute, but I tell arthritis patients that it won't work well for them. It has no anti-inflammatory properties, which is part of the value of aspirin. Another drawback is that if it is overused, it can harm the liver.

An interesting product made from acetaminophen and antihistamine is Percogesic. The acetaminophen relieves pain, and the antihistamine relaxes muscles, which is a great help with some muscle conditions. But it can make you drowsy. (See side effects for antihistamine products in Chapter 2.)

Back to aspirin, for people with no special problems, I recommend the less expensive brands because they are all alike. Aspirin is also very popular in combination products, which often contain aspirin, acetaminophen and caffeine. Excedrin is one of those products. It gives me my best headache relief. If I take half a tablet, I get relief from a normal headache in fifteen minutes.

I disapprove when people consume excessive amounts of caffeine merely to control their diet or to force themselves to stay awake intemperately, but I think caffeine is well justified in pain medications. Obviously, if you begin to need five or six aspirin tablets to deal with a normal headache, such use is no longer justified, and your doctor should be consulted for assistance.

The exciting news in over-the-counter analgesics now is ibuprofen, which you can buy as Advil, Nuprin and Medipren. Ibuprofen may be more effective than aspirin and helps relieve arthritis, toothache and backache. And it is especially good for menstrual cramps. It fights inflammation and swelling as well as pain. When you buy ibuprofen with a prescription, you get it in 400-, 600- or 800-milligram doses. When you buy it over the counter, you get it in 200-milligram doses. Like aspirin, ibuprofen can upset the stomach and is best taken with food.

I have designed a chart to summarize the facts about these basic analgesics:

ANALGESICS

Product and Ingredients	When to Use	Side Effects and Warnings
Aspirin Bayer Norwich Aspirin Many other brands *(Ingredients: Acetylsalicylic acid, (ASA))*	General analgesic purposes; reduces pain, fever; relieves joint pain, swelling or stiffness	Stomach upset, Reye's syndrome, negative interaction with other medicines or ringing in ears; consult doctor first, if you have asthma, gout or stomach or duodenal ulcers

Product	When to Use	Side Effects and Warnings
Coated Aspirin Ecotrin *(Ingredients:* *Acetylsalicylic acid,* *(ASA))*	Same as above, but use this product when aspirin upsets stomach or when large amounts are needed for chronic or long-term pain relief	Reye's syndrome, negative interaction with other medicines; stop usage if you have dizziness, ringing in ears or loss of hearing; check with your doctor if you have an aspirin-sensitive disease
Buffered Aspirin Ascriptin Bufferin *(Ingredients: Coated* *aspirin (ASA) with* *antacid)*	Same as above	See above side effects and warnings
Combination Products Excedrin *(Ingredients: Aspirin* *(ASA), acetaminophen,* *caffeine* BC Powder *(Ingredients: Aspirin* *(ASA), salicylamide,* *caffeine)* Anacin *(Ingredients: Aspirin* *(ASA), caffeine)* Vanquish *(Ingredients: Aspirin* *(ASA), acetaminophen,* *caffeine, antacid)*	These usually contain small amounts of caffeine, which add a stimulant effect (or a sense of well being). Use for colds, flu, headache, muscular aches, menstrual cramps or sinusitis	Stomach upset, can cause jitters; see above side effects; check each product for warnings
Acetaminophen Anacin-3 Datril Panadol Infants' Tylenol* Children's Tylenol* Junior Strength Tylenol* Generic brands *(Ingredients:* *Acetaminophen)*	Use as a substitute for aspirin, especially for infants, children or teenagers, to prevent Reye's syndrome; use for fever, headaches, minor aches and pains	Not anti-inflammatory; can harm liver after long use or large doses

Product	When to Use	Side Effects and Warnings
Ibuprofen Advil* Nuprin Medipren *(Ingredients:* *Ibuprofen)*	Use for arthritis, cold, headache, menstrual cramps, minor back and joint inflammation or toothache	Check pregnancy warnings; check with your doctor if you are taking any prescription drugs or if you have had any side effects from non-prescription pain relievers before taking ibuprofen; see a doctor if you have any symptoms that are unusual or unrelated to your original ailment; do not take this drug with other ibuprofen products or any other pain reliever.

*I use or recommend

No one can guess what great improvements might be added to this chart in the future. Researchers are at work on potent, non-addictive painkillers that will probably become available through prescription before long, and we can expect new over-the-counter spinoffs.

Worth Remembering

A desire to take medicine is, perhaps, the great feature which distinguishes man from other animals.
—*Sir William Osler*[3]

GETTING THE MOST OUT OF A DOCTOR'S APPOINTMENT

Visiting a doctor's office is an intimidating experience for many people. Remember, the doctor is there to serve you. You are the one who is feeling sick, and you have the right to ask any question related to your symptoms and the subsequent diagnosis. If your doctor is unwilling to spend the time to answer your questions, consider changing doctors.

Of course, the doctor can't operate in a vacuum. You must be as clear, concise and descriptive as possible when explaining your symptoms. Don't be afraid to mention details you think may be insignificant—those little details may provide the key that unlocks the entire problem.

Sometimes it may even be helpful to jot your symptoms on a slip of paper before you visit your doctor. That way you won't inadvertently forget to mention an important point because you're nervous or you feel rushed. The more facts you provide your doctor, the easier it is for him or her to provide an accurate diagnosis.

It's vitally important to inform a new doctor or remind your regular doctor about your medical history. Don't expect your doctor to remember. He or she has a lot of patients. Mention previous diagnoses, prescribed medications and what side effects you may have experienced.

Let your doctor know what medications you are presently taking. This is important for two reasons. First, medication can mask symptoms. For instance, if you take a Tylenol or an aspirin an hour before you meet with your doctor, you will probably show a lower fever—or no fever—when the doctor takes your temperature.

Second, certain medications can interfere with the effectiveness of other medications; in fact, certain combinations can be lethal. By knowing what you are presently taking, the doctor can avoid prescribing any medication that could produce dangerous complications.

After the doctor has listened to your symptoms and history and has suggested a possible diagnosis, don't be afraid to ask questions about the pathology (that is, the nature of the disease or disorder) which has been diagnosed.

Suppose your doctor told you that you have high blood pressure. Of course, most of us have heard of high blood pressure, but even though it's commonly known, be certain you really know what it is.

Once you know the diagnosis, here are some questions you could ask the doctor:
—What does it really mean?
—How will it impact my life?
—What normally happens to someone who has it?
—Can I get over it?
—What can you do to treat it?

Don't hesitate to ask your doctor to repeat anything you don't understand. Remember, it is your body and your life. You deserve to understand what's happening to you, and the doctor is the expert to help you do just that.

After you fully understand the nature of your problem, explore with your doctor the various courses of treatment available to deal with your situation. If the doctor simply prescribes one particular course of treatment, ask about other options. Have him or her explain the pros and cons of each option. While it is true that the doctor is the expert, you should have the right to make an intelligent assessment of the various options since it's your life that is being affected.

When a course of treatment has been decided on, the doctor should carefully explain the various reactions you can expect along the way, the possible side effects and the length of treatment. It's easy for a doctor to get so caught up in the busyness of the day, the thirty patients out in the waiting room, the hospital emergency that kept him or her up all night, or some minor staffing personnel problem, that he or she may neglect to fully explain your treatment to you. Simply keep asking questions until you are sure you understand what the doctor is trying to accomplish by the treatment prescribed. Any doctor who is unwilling to provide a reasonable amount of time for an explanation is probably not a doctor with whom you will remain happy.

It's my personal conviction that if you fully understand the nature of the problem from which you suffer and if you fully understand how the doctor plans to treat it, the healing process will be greatly enhanced. You'll leave the doctor's office with more confidence.

Despite a meaningful visit with the doctor, however, you can still be confused when the doctor hands you a prescription to take to a drugstore. If you try to figure it out, you can't make head nor tail of it. It might as well be written in another language. Deciphering that prescription is discussed in the next chapter.

Worth Remembering

I treated him, God cured him.
—*Ambroise Pare's favorite saying* [1]

PRESCRIPTIONS AND HOW TO READ THEM

As you puzzle over the prescription in your hand, one of the first items you'll ponder is a mysterious Rx mark. Most people assume it's some difficult medical term. But it just means "recipe." (No"x" is used in our word "recipe," but the old Latin word has one.)

Every prescription from a doctor is a kind of recipe within a recipe. First, it has directions for the pharmacist to follow; second, it includes directions for the pharmacist to pass on to the patient. (It's best if the doctor tells the directions to the patient and the pharmacist repeats them to the patient as well as putting them on the label.)

Nowadays the pharmacist fills a prescription by simply following a careful "lick, stick, count and pour" routine. He or she accurately fills and labels vials and bottles from a supply of manufactured medicines. But in the old days, pharmacists had to prepare a lot of medications from the raw products, grinding and mixing according to doctors' directions. It was rather like a cook following a recipe to make a chemical stew of one kind or another.

Today pharmacists are much better trained in diagnosis and bioavailability (the factors affecting the drug when it enters the body). They also know the positive and the adverse effects to expect from drugs, plus other factors that can influence a course of treatment with medication.

Patients can rarely read the notes they take to the pharmacy for two reasons. First, doctors write in a kind of secret code that only medical people bother to learn. Second, doctors tend to scribble. As a result, even patients who want to know as much as possible tend to feel mystified by the writing on their prescriptions and end up simply trusting their doctor and pharmacist.

That's usually a safe course of action, but I can think of one exception to that. One day a woman came to my counter with a question. She handed me her vial of pills and asked why she was extremely drowsy since starting to take them a few days earlier.

Glancing at the label, I saw that the vial contained Doriden and that she was instructed to take one tablet at bedtime. Doriden is a strong sleeping potion used for insomnia. I looked up the original prescription in my file; it called for just what was on the label. I asked the woman the nature of the medical problem for which her physician was treating her.

"I was constipated, and he prescribed a laxative," the woman answered.

After examining the prescription again, I finally figured out what must have happened. The physician had forgotten to cross the *x* in the word *Doxidan,* and so it seemed to spell Doriden. (Doxidan is a laxative.)

I excused myself, hurried to the telephone, called the doctor and told him what had happened. He burst into laughter and told me not to worry, that the woman didn't really need a laxative anyway and that maybe the extra sleep did her some good. Fortunately, this kind of misunderstanding is rare.

Some people wish there were new rules for the way prescriptions are written. They could be in plain English, for instance, or doctors could have little prescription-writing machines that would print the words clearly. Illegible handwriting by doctors is an old joke that the public tolerates with good humor.

But I think the public believes that we pharmacists are trained to read bad handwriting. Believe me, we aren't; we can't read it any better than anyone else. We often have to call the doctors to find out what a prescription is supposed to say.

And we aren't the only ones with that problem. Nurses sometimes misread doctors' instructions. Once a nurse put ear drops into a hospital patient's rectum because the doctor's scribble for "right ear" seemed to say "rear."

In case you're interested and your doctor writes legibly enough, here is a guide for your prescriptions (doctors may write abbreviations in capital or lower case letters):

PRESCRIPTION CODE INTERPRETATION

	Code	Interpretation
Amounts	ī	one
	īī	two
	īīī	three
	īv̄	four
	v̄	five
	x̄	ten
	L	fifty
	C	hundred
	ss̄	half
	ʒī	one teaspoonful
	ʒīī	two teaspoonfuls

	Code	**Interpretation**
Amounts (cont.)	℥ss	half teaspoonful
	mg.	milligram
	gm	gram
	gms	grams
	gr	grain
	grs	grains
	#1	1/8 grain, or 7.5 milligrams
	#2	1/4 grain, or 15 milligrams
	#3	1/2 grain, or 30 milligrams
	#4	1 grain, or 60 milligrams
	TAB	tablet
	CAP	capsule
	GTT	drop
	GTTS	drops
	oz.	ounce
Timing	PRN	as needed
	HS	at bedtime
	PC	after meals
	AC	before meals
	Q	every
	D or QD	every day
	BID	twice a day
	TID	three times a day
	QID	four times a day
	QW	once a week
	BIW	twice a week
	TIW	three times a week
	QIW	four times a week
	QOD	every other day
Body Parts	OU	both eyes
	OS	left eye
	OD	right eye
	AU	both ears
	AS	left ear
	AD	right ear
	PV or VAG	vaginally
	PR	rectally
	OTIC	ear
	OPTH	eye
	PO	orally

	Code	Interpretation
Directions	SIG	directions
	UD	as directed
	APP	applicator
	X	multiplication sign

Following are some sample prescriptions as they are typically written in the above code, while the directions are explained in plain English underneath.

AJ1103567
G3056

JOHN D. JOME, M.D.
1435 SOUTH ST.
PASADENA, CA 91107

NAME: _____ DATE: _____

ADDRESS: _____

TELEPHONE: _____

Tetracycline 250 mg. #40
SIG ī QID

REFILL: _____

LABEL: _____   _____

Tetracycline 250 mg. #40
SIG ī QID
One capsule four times a day.

```
AJ1103567                    JOHN D. JOME, M.D.
G3056                           1435 SOUTH ST.
                             PASADENA, CA 91107

NAME: _____  DATE: _____

ADDRESS: _____

TELEPHONE: _____

  Auralgan otic drops
  SIG iii GTTS AU TID


REFILL: _____
LABEL: _____       _____
```

Auralgan otic drops
SIG ӥ GTTS AU TID
Three drops into both ears three times a day

```
AJ1103567                    JOHN D. JOME, M.D.
G3056                           1435 SOUTH ST.
                             PASADENA, CA 91107

NAME: _____  DATE: _____

ADDRESS: _____

TELEPHONE: _____

  Phenergan with Codeine
  6oz.
  SIG ʒi TID PRN Cough
REFILL: _____
LABEL: _____       _____
```

Phenergan with Codeine
6 oz.
SIG ʒi TID PRN Cough
Take one teaspoonful three times a day as needed for cough

AJ1103567
G3056

JOHN D. JOME, M.D.
1435 SOUTH ST.
PASADENA, CA 91107

NAME: _____ DATE: _____

ADDRESS: _____

TELEPHONE: _____

Tylenol #3

#30

SIG ī or īī Q 3-4 hrs PRN pain

REFILL: _____

LABEL: _____   _____

Tylenol #3

#30

SIG ī or īī Q 3-4 hrs PRN pain

Take one or two tablets every 3-4 hours as needed for pain

AJ1103567
G3056

JOHN D. JOME, M.D.
1435 SOUTH ST.
PASADENA, CA 91107

NAME: _____ DATE: _____

ADDRESS: _____

TELEPHONE: _____

Monistat vag cream.

45 gms

SIG ī APP PV QHS X 7D

REFILL: _____

LABEL: _____   _____

Monistat vag cream

45 gms

SIG ī APP PV QHS X 7D

Insert one applicatorful vaginally every bedtime for 7 days

```
AJ1103567                    JOHN D. JOME, M.D.
G3056                           1435 SOUTH ST.
                              PASADENA, CA 91107

NAME: _____  DATE: _____

ADDRESS: _____

TELEPHONE: _____

    Donnatal Tabs
    SIG ss̄ TID AC+ HS

REFILL: _____
LABEL: _____            _____
```

Donnatal Tabs
SIG s̄s̄ TID AC + HS
Take 1/2 tablet three times a day before meals and at bedtime

Another help for decoding prescriptions is knowing where to look on the page for certain information. Prescriptions are usually arranged in the same general pattern. In the left-hand corner is the drug enforcement number and below that the state license number. Below these numbers is the patient's name, address and age, and the date of the prescription. In the middle appears the name of the medication with its strength, and under that the number of doses the doctor is prescribing.

Directly beneath that are the directions for the patient that the pharmacist translates into English and gives to the patient. Near the lower-left corner is the number of refills that the doctor allows. (For some drugs there is a time limit on when the refills can be made, but this information is not included on the prescription form.) Near the lower-right corner the physician signs his or her name. Under the name is a space for the doctor's registered number for use when prescribing addictive medications. Here is the typical prescription format:

Drug enforcement administration number State license number	JOHN D. BROWN, M.D. 210 NORTH ST. POMONA, CA 91768	
Patient's name		Date
Patient's address		Patient's age
	Medication Quantity	
SIG: Directions to be given to the patient		
Number of refills		Doctor's signature
(Doctor's address is here or at the top.)		Doctor's registered number

Limits on prescription refills are set to try to keep people from intentionally or accidentally increasing their dosage. In California, doctors often prescribe controlled medications this way: "Five refills or six months, whichever comes first." For less dangerous medications, such as thyroid supplements, I have seen prescriptions on which the doctor authorized one hundred refills or "refills forever." But it's the responsibility of the pharmacist to call and check with the doctor at least once a year.

Limited refills serve as a protection for the doctor and for the patient when pharmacists make sure prescriptions are up to date. A patient could justifiably sue both doctor and pharmacist for being too lax on long-term prescriptions.

In one drugstore where I worked, I found that some prescriptions had been refilled for years without being checked. I called to verify them with the prescribing physician and in several cases I was told, "I didn't know I still had that person for a patient."

One patient had been buying refills of Proloid, a thyroid medication, for twelve years on an old prescription. I called the doctor to check and discovered that the doctor was dead.

You may wonder why it sometimes takes so long to get your prescription refilled. On occasion, your pharmacist needs to call the doctor to confirm it's okay to refill the prescription. If you request your refill at 5 P.M. on Thursday and your doctor has left the office already and takes Friday off, you won't be able to have your prescription filled until Monday. In some cases, a pharmacist can give you four or five tablets to get you by until he or she can reach the doctor.

When I worked in a drugstore in Lancaster, California, a local doctor was notorious for not responding to our calls. A patient would call in the morning to order a refill, and we would call the doctor's office and wait for a return call.

In the afternoon, the patient would come in for the medication, and we would call the doctor's office again. The nurse would answer that he had not yet responded to the notes on his desk, so the prescription was not cleared. I would usually give the patient a tablet or two and tell him or her to check back the next day. This went on and on. The doctor was always busy or out of the office.

Once when I made a repeat call, I said, "This is the pharmacy, and you can forget the prescription for Ian Brady. He has a heart problem and is now lying on the floor here!"

That time the doctor himself was on the phone in twenty seconds, demanding, "What happened to Brady? Is he all right? Did you call the paramedics?"

I said, "Doctor, I am the pharmacist who has been calling you for three days trying to get you to okay your prescription for Mr. Brady."

The doctor was absolutely furious, but he did okay the prescription.

In reality, 90 percent of doctors' offices return prescription calls promptly.

Another fact many people don't know is that some medications have special rules. In most states, you have to get certain prescriptions filled within seven days or else they expire. And certain medications like Percodan or Percocet or Paregoric require special triplicate prescriptions because the drugs are addictive. Doctors can order those by telephone for you only in case of an emergency. Then they must mail in a handwritten prescription form within seventy-two hours for the pharmacy records.

"Scrip doctors" run prescription mills, writing out prescriptions for thirty or sixty pills such as Empirin with Codeine (that acts like morphene) or Preludin (appetite suppressants). The "patients" would pay the doctors twenty-five or thirty dollars whenever they went in for a prescription. The doctors keep "charts" but never examine the patients. The patients either take all the pills themselves or sell them for about triple what they paid.

After a while, I wouldn't fill prescriptions from downtown Los Angeles; I said that we dealt only with local doctors in our suburb. One day two men came in with a prescription from a local doctor, but I didn't trust them. I called the doctor to check and learned that the prescription was forged. Next I called the police. The men were still sitting there waiting for their drugs when the police arrested them.

The men I turned in didn't give me any trouble, but sometimes pharmacists are in danger. In fact, a pharmacist I knew was shot and killed after he had gone to court to testify against a drug user. As soon as the court put the man on probation, he went back to the pharmacy and killed the pharmacist who had turned him in.

One of the saddest drug incidents I dealt with involved a young man named Jedd, who came limping in with a triplicate prescription for Percodan from a local doctor. He told me how he had been injured, and I took quite a liking to him. He came back in two or three weeks for a refill and told me about the ankle surgery he was going to have. He came in about once a month for about ten months, always at the right time for his medication, never early. He usually brought me up to date about his grandmother in Seattle and his business. At one point, his doctor changed him to a different pain medication that didn't require the triplicate prescription.

One day that doctor called me, and I happened to ask, "By the way, you have a patient named Jedd Smith, don't you?"

I was shocked when he said no. I pride myself on being able to spot a forgery, but I had been tricked by the triplicate form, which is hard to forge, and the good manners of this clean-cut young man. I wished he would never return.

But in a few weeks, in he walked as usual. I told him that I was all out of that medication and would have the prescription ready for him the next day. Then I contacted the police, and they told me to call them as soon as he came back in for his medication.

The next day he came in and told me that he had recently been to Seattle to put his grandmother into a nursing home. While we were chatting, my assistant called the police. Jedd thanked me and walked out the door with his medication as usual.

Just then about six police cars zoomed up from all directions, and the police grabbed Jedd a few doors up the street. They looked into the trunk of his car and found a small drugstore there—empty bottles from various local pharmacies, several forged prescriptions and pads of blank forms. Their first concern, of course, was that he might be selling the drugs.

When Jedd related his story, it was discovered that he had been in a bad swimming-pool accident several years earlier, that had smashed his face and broken several bones. By the time the surgeries were over, Jedd was addicted to pain medication. He tried a treatment program, but it didn't work. After he was arrested, he decided to try again. I hope he succeeded.

Generic or Name Brand?

One of the biggest questions people have about their prescriptions today is whether they should purchase generic drugs instead of name brand drugs. Unless a doctor indicates on the prescription that a certain name brand is required, the patient and pharmacist can choose.

The main reason for considering generics is financial. Patients pay much less for generic drugs, and pharmacists usually increase their profits, so both parties benefit. The active ingredients in generic and brand-name drugs are supposed to be exactly the same, although the fillers and binders differ. Most patients do just as well with generic antibiotics, cold and allergy products, arthritis medications, pain medications and high blood pressure medications as they do with the brand-name forms.

Fifty-nine firms make brand-name drugs, and they dominate the market in prescription drugs. They are the ones who do the chemical research and the expensive advertising to launch the product, and so they need a return on their investment. For ten years or more, they have exclusive control over their products.

But when the patent expires, other companies can apply to the government for permission to produce and market that same medicine under its noncommercial name. (Thus a Valium prescription that costs $27.47 can be replaced by a Diazepam prescription that costs only $8.49, now produced by more than a dozen companies.) One study showed that a savings of twenty-five percent, or close to $4 billion, in 1981 could have been passed on to the consumer if generic instead of brand-name drugs had been bought.[1]

Customers certainly don't want to buy substitute medications from dirty or careless companies that produce them cheaply. But 80 percent of generic drugs are produced by the name-brand drug companies themselves,[2] and the producers of the other 20 percent are answerable to the Food and Drug Administration.

I'm aware of some questions that have been raised recently about the content of generic medications and, as this book goes to press, the FDA is investigating scattered violations by generic manufacturers. My personal experience with generic drugs has generally been positive; I've encountered few problems.

One exception is with the product Premarin. I personally like to use most generics, but I advise my patients who use Premarin, a hormone drug, to stick with the original because it is more reliable and gives better results.

Most patients have good results if they switch to generics. But you should check with your doctor about your particular medications and should also make it a point to notice any changes that might occur after the switch. Even the difference in binders can have an influence on some people.

Incidentally, many people assume that medicines that have to be purchased by prescription are more powerful or more dangerous than medicines purchased over the counter. That's not always the case. The line between prescription and over-the-counter medicine is often arbitrary and rather hazy. Many items could go either way, and indeed they sometimes cross over the line as times change.

Some people want fewer and fewer products to require prescriptions, and others want to require prescriptions even for vitamins.

The manufacturers' desires are one major factor in those decisions; they prefer to market some of their products one way and some another way as part of their business strategy. We end up with a compromise situation in which the decisions are not entirely consistent, but overall the system works well.

Needless to say, when prescription medications are used, the doctor is in the position of authority. When over-the-counter medications are used, the doctor might be left out of the picture altogether—although I don't think that's a good idea.

The pharmacist can be a big help when it comes to making over-the-counter decisions since he or she has had to take many classes that are similar to those doctors take. During pharmacy school, a student spends two to four months acquiring field experience, called rotation, in nursing homes, pharmacies and hospitals. Some states actually require a whole year of this kind of experience before a Doctorate of Pharmacy is issued to a student.

During my rotation, I had opportunities to handle medication, fill prescriptions and observe surgeries. My field experience occurred in a county hospital in Omaha, Nebraska, where I attended pharmacy school.

At that county hospital, the morning began with a team of ten to twelve doctors and student interns studying X-rays and making rounds. The afternoon was spent attending lectures, collecting histories from patients and observing surgery.

One morning our medical entourage entered a patient's room. As we gathered around the bed, the doctor looked at us and said, "This gentleman is presenting a high fever and a possible gall bladder situation. What is your recommendation?"

With trepidation, we carefully studied the facts. Directly in front of us lay the patient whose life depended on our rather neophyte prescriptive skills.

At last I mustered up enough courage to suggest possible treatment. I waited to get shot down by the chief resident. To my surprise and relief, he agreed. That marked an awesome and wonderful moment for me. I realized that what I had learned in pharmacy school was being translated into reality.

We also learned from our mistakes on rotation. Once I filled a prescription for a drug called Compazine, which came in both tablets and capsules. I simply chose to use the tablets. I was wrong. My supervisor directed me back to the prescription. It read: "Take one every twelve hours." Twelve hours obviously called for a time release, which only the capsules provided.

I was devastated by this error. I had to remind myself that it was better to make an error under supervision and learn from my mistakes at that point rather than later when I would no longer have the benefit of supervision. I also began to build safeguards into my work, such as a triple-check safety system. Like other pharmacists, I had to pass a rigorous state exam before I ever received my pharmaceutical license.

After graduation, I realized the pharmacist has the responsibility to make sure the customer understands what medication he or she is taking and how to administer it correctly. Otherwise, dangerous repercussions can occur.

One of my regular customers, Mr. Sinquist, had taken heart medication daily for several years. One day, he came in to tell me he had been sick. After asking him several questions, I realized why he had become so ill. He had decided that if one of those heart pills made him feel good, then surely two or three would make him feel better.

"Mr. Sinquist," I began, determined not to sound panicked. "By taking more than the doctor prescribed, do you realize you have been poisoning yourself?"

Once I explained to him how his medication worked, he knew he would never make the same mistake again. As a further reminder, Mr. Sinquist's physician took him off the pills completely so his body could recover.

Another way of diverting any possible disaster is to make sure your pharmacist is as aware of your history as your family doctor. That's why you should consistently go to the same pharmacy and get to know the pharmacist. Many pharmacies are now keeping track of an individual's medications by computer.

I don't know how many times I've asked a question like, "Mrs. Jones, you aren't allergic to penicillin, are you?"

"Oh, yes, I am. But it's on my doctor's chart. He knows."

"Well, there's a slipup. This antibiotic is a form of penicillin. I'll call your doctor right now to see what he wants to do."

In a sense, the pharmacist often plays the role of a counselor. It's not unusual for a pharmacist to deal with people who are terminally ill. I can usually tell just from reading the prescription that the person is dying. As each week goes by, I watch death's grip tighten on that body. At such times, I believe God wants me to take the time to interact with the person and learn about his or her fears. I truly see pharmacy as a ministry, a place where hope is offered.

In his book *The Healing of Persons,* Dr. Paul Tournier told about the importance of dispensing hope as well as medications. He had a sickly patient named Benjamin who had been a walking nervous breakdown ever since his only child died long ago. He rarely contacted his wife but spent his life going from one clinic to another, looking for physical help for his digestive troubles and general misery.

Dr. Tournier finally confronted Benjamin and told him that what he really needed was to turn to Christ. He needed to accept what came to him, carry his cross in life, put up with troubles, go back to work and face up to life's hurts. Dr. Tournier assured the man that Christ would be at his side if he did so and that such a life has joy in it.

Benjamin saw that Tournier was right, but he didn't know how to change. Dr. Tournier took out his prescription pad and handed it to Benjamin. "We are going to listen to God together, and you must write down what he says to you," Dr. Tournier ordered.

After a while Benjamin wrote: "I am ill because I think of nothing but myself. I must do some loving action."

That very day he wrote to his wife for the first time in three months and told her that he had found God. He expressed affection for her, asked for her forgiveness and said he hoped to return, go back to work and make her happy. At supper that evening he was in high spirits and surprised everyone with his good appetite. He was on the road to recovery.[3]

Worth Remembering

Rx—Prayer, as needed, for all of life.

—K. L.

THE WELL-STOCKED MEDICINE CABINET

Most Americans would be shocked, should they ever clean out their medicine cabinets, to discover such a funny mixture of old things collected there. They are not alone. Even pharmacists, who should know better, have an embarrassing old clutter in the medicine cabinet.

We are going to enter the inner sanctum of my own bathroom. Today I have decided to do what all people should do at least once a year—clean out the medicine cabinet. In the process, I'm going to explain what every well-stocked medicine cabinet ought to have—and what it ought not to have.

Let's start at the top. First I take down a small box that contains a sample bottle of Neo-Synephrine (0.25%) nose drops for children. No date is on the bottle. Judging by the dust on the box, I would guess that it's at least three years old. If an item has no date and you don't know its age, toss it out. I pour the few drops of liquid into the sink.

Next, I take down a sample one-ounce bottle of Tylenol that expired six years ago! Into the sink with it. Toss only empty vials and bottles that have been rinsed out into the wastebasket. You never know when children might get into the trash, play with your medicine bottles and eat or drink the ingredients.

The Tylenol reminds me of a time when we were visiting friends, and my daughter started getting a headache after bumping her head. I asked our friends if they had any Tylenol. They brought me two kinds to choose from: extra-strength caplets (more than a normal adult dose) and liquid. I checked the directions on the liquid and gave my daughter the proper dose for a child. Then I noticed that the Tylenol had expired more than a year before! The medicine cabinet seems to be a graveyard of expired medications.

What ought a well-stocked medicine cabinet contain? I would suggest the following, then we'll continue the tour of my own medicine cabinet, which is full of other lessons on what to do and not to do with those medications.

The Well-Stocked Medicine Cabinet

Pain Relief
1. Aspirin or combination:
   Bayer
   Bufferin
   Excedrin
2. Tylenol
   Panadol
   or
   Datril
3. Ibuprofen
   Advil

Nuprin
or
Store brand
4. Bandages and tapes:
Box of assorted bandages
2" Ace bandage
2" x 2" gauze pads
1" rolled gauze
1/2" adhesive tape
Box of butterfly bandages (medium)
5. Actifed Tablets or Actifed Syrup
6. Benylin, Delsym or Robitussin-DM
7. Chloraseptic Lozenges (also spray) or Halls Mentho-Lyptus
8. Collyrium for Fresh Eyes wash or Prefrin Liquifilm eye drops
9. Donnagel liquid (Kaopectate for young children) or Lomotil (by prescription only)
10. Mylanta, Riopan or other antacid
11. Neosporin ointment, Hibiclens or hydrogen peroxide
12. Foille ointment
13. Balmex Ointment or hydrocortisone 0.5% cream (many companies)
14. Thermometer
15. If you need a sleep aid: Benadryl (antihistamine used as a sleep aid) or Sominex (with diphenhydramine)
16. If you need a laxative: Metamucil, Effer-Syllium (first choice)

Now, back to my medicine cabinet. Here's a product I prize—a bottle of Lomotil tablets. This is the best prescription for diarrhea from viral flu or food poisoning; one or two doses usually does the trick. Lomotil is just the thing to take on a trip to a foreign country where the water may upset your intestines. (You have to plan ahead so you can get it through your doctor before your trip.) I see that this bottle has nine tablets left, enough to cover a couple of days of diarrhea. It's good for two more years, so I'll keep it.

I remember how I woke up with diarrhea about three in the morning one time and hurried to the medicine cabinet and opened the Lomotil bottle. All that was left was powder; the tablets had disintegrated. I figured out that my addiction to long, hot showers had taken its toll on the Lomotil.

If you can draw little pictures in the condensed steam on the cabinet mirror, you know that the products inside are getting a moist-heat treatment also. Should that description sound like your bathroom, I would suggest storing medications in a hall closet or a bedroom drawer. (Always remember that it's important to store medications out of the reach of small children.)

Here's another bottle of Lomotil tablets, and this one doesn't expire for three more years. I can imagine tidy folk dumping tablets from one of these bottles into the other to save shelf space. Don't do that! Keep medication with different expiration dates in separate containers.

I'm often asked how long medication is still good after the expiration date. I'd say that six months is questionable. I wouldn't use any medication two years after the expiration date. Some medications like aspirin can break down into harmful products that might make the user sick. At best, outdated medicines are apt to be no help to you. Before you buy a product, always check the expiration date. Don't assume that everything is current and fresh on the shelves.

Next, I discover a Valium prescription. This is one of the most notorious medicines of our time. It was the most popular drug of the 1970s, and was prescribed for everything from job stress to widowhood, from back pain to heroin withdrawal. Valium made a fortune for the Hoffman-La Roche company, and then horror stories started coming out about the damage done by overuse and addiction.

We have a bottle in our medicine cabinet because, when we lived in La Verne, California, we rented a house beside an open field. We were besieged by black widow spiders.

One morning I woke up at about 2 A.M. with incredible burning in my leg, as if someone had jammed a hot poker into the back of my thigh. I hobbled into the bathroom and saw a huge red spot on my leg.

I went back to the bed and pulled down the covers, but I was staring bleary-eyed at our favorite sheets, a leopard-print design with inky black spots everywhere. Believe it or not, in the midst of all those black spots I saw one black spot that was a dead spider. I examined it and discovered it was a black widow. I had no idea what to do for such a poison bite.

I went to the emergency room of my local hospital. By the time I got there, my thigh was hot, and my groin was swollen and cramping. The doctor told me that he wouldn't give me any antivenom if he could avoid it, because it can cause problems itself. So he monitored my blood pressure and gave me a Valium for the muscle spasms in my leg. It worked great. I took it one or two more times in the next week to ease my discomfort. But that was long ago, and this Valium is expired. I toss the tablets into the toilet.

Next, I pull down a bottle of ophthalmic solution, which is no longer in its original box with the directions on it. If you get the old eye infection and run to the medicine cabinet for the drops, the scene might go something like this: "Ah, there it is, right behind the shaving cream. Now, how was I supposed to use this? No instructions. Oh well, I'll just squirt some in." Keep the prescription label, expiration date and directions for every medication until you throw the medication away. The eye drops are obviously expired, as well as lacking directions, so out they go.

Here is Donnagel, which I recommend for diarrhea and stomach cramps. All over-the-counter items have a date on them now, so this one is very old indeed because it has no date. Out it goes.

Here is my soft, blue bottle of Hibiclens, an antimicrobial cleanser that the emergency room doctors used on me after I received some minor cuts in a recent accident. Hydrogen peroxide is the old standby cleanser, but I think some of the new products like Phresh 3.5, Hibiclens and Betadine Skin Cleanser are worth having in the medicine cabinet.

People sometimes come in and ask me for "the skin cleanser that comes in the square yellow bottle." That one is Betadine. Our most popular brand of antibacterial cleanser used to be pHisoHex, but it contained the antiseptic hexachlorophene—which was in almost four hundred products, including toothpaste, soap, shampoo, skin cream, mouthwash, lip pomade, deodorant and baby powder.

Hexachlorophene was such a fad ingredient that at its height of popularity you couldn't find any kind of lip balm that didn't include it. In many hospitals, new babies were washed with it. In 1972, it was discovered that hexachlorophene was toxic, that it was absorbed through the skin, and caused brain damage in infants. Now, pHisoHex is distributed by prescription only, and if you ever come across an old, bright green bottle of pHisoHex, check with your physician before using it.

My next bottle is a sample of Sudafed Cough Syrup, a fairly good product. But for children I prefer Actifed Syrup because it has an antihistamine, is an excellent ear decongestant and makes kids drowsy. (Check with your doctor before giving Actifed or Sudafed to kids six or under. Sometimes they cause excitability or make them a bit hyperactive.) This particular bottle of Sudafed has no expiration date, so out it goes. By the way, this sample did not have a safety cap. Either make sure that bottles without safety caps are too high for the children to reach or else put them under lock and key somewhere.

Safety caps can be frustrating, but they prevent about three hundred children's deaths every year. Protective caps are well worth the trouble. Nevertheless, some children can open any safety cap, and some adults can't open any of them.

One day an extremely frustrated woman about seventy-five-years old came up to my counter. I could see trouble in her eyes as she approached me.

"May I help you?" I asked.

"Yes, can you get this darned safety cap off?" she asked, as she trembled. She held up a twisted plastic vial full of pills, with the safety cap in place. I asked her what in the world had happened.

"I couldn't get the cap off, and I needed my medicine," she explained. "I took the bottle to my neighbor, and he couldn't get the top off. So he got his hammer, and we tried to break it off. We couldn't."

I got the cap off and poured her pills into a new vial with a regular cap. Anyone who wants a regular cap can get one by asking. A regular cap can be worth a thousand dollars to the adult who can't remove the top to get the pills out of the bottle.

Here's an old bottle of Kaopectate, which I don't use anymore. This dusty old bottle is almost full, but it expired in 1984. As I pour it down the sink, I notice that only clear liquid comes out because the medicine has settled at the bottom. It needs shaking. If anyone tries to take Kaopectate in the dark, he or she might get just the liquid off the top of it.

My next discovery is a bottle of Regular Strength Tylenol that is sealed and has an expiration date well in the future. People should always have good pain relievers on hand for those little emergencies like toothaches, leg cramps and menstrual cramps.

Every medicine cabinet should contain aspirin or some other favorite headache remedy, plus an ibuprofen product for severe pain. Here's my old bottle of Nuprin.

One morning last year I rolled over in bed and felt deep pain in my shoulder. This was the Fourth of July weekend, so it would be four days before I could see an orthopedic doctor. I started to take two Nuprin tablets three times a day with food. When I finally got to see a doctor, the bursitis was starting to loosen up, but my Nuprin had seen me through a long weekend.

Looking into the Nuprin bottle, I find its yellow tablets mixed with a few white tablets. They are Excedrin analgesic tablets. I am not going to name names, but obviously someone in this family has mixed the medications. I realize this is a handy way to take familiar pills along on a trip. But medications should be kept separate and properly labelled to avoid mistakes.

Next is a bottle with four antibiotic tablets in it. They are left over from when my wife had some dental surgery last year, and they have expired now. Ordinarily, you should throw away leftover drugs as soon as you finish with them. Don't save them for someone else to use.

People should never share prescription medicine with each other, even in the same family. Every family member's illness should be diagnosed separately by a doctor, and a new prescription should be written for each family member. This keeps the doctor informed and in charge.

Next is a bottle from Hawaiian Tropic with aloe vera in it, which is our favorite product for preventing sunburn. It also has lidocaine in it to deaden pain. But it looks old and the color has changed, so I'll throw it out.

Now I see something more difficult to throw away, a small spray can of Dermoplast anesthetic, and it looks old. It isn't safe to throw a usable spray can into the trash. Roll up the can in a trash bag, tape the bag shut, seal it in a box and write "toxic" on the box. It's also a good idea to take the can outside and spray it until it's empty before throwing it away.

Here is a small bottle of Excedrin P.M., a nighttime pain reliever. Thank goodness that doctors are backing off now from the narcotic sleeping aids that have so often been more of a harm than a help to people. Fewer people are using Seconal Sodium or Tuinal for insomnia, and that's good. It's ironic that some of the medications people have used for insomnia really increase the insomnia in the long run, so the more they take, the more they seem to need the pills. I call this "insomnia rebound."

Sleeping aids used to contain pyrilamine maleate, but that drug may increase the risk of cancer and is far less common now. Today's sleep aids are more apt to contain diphenhydramine hydrochloride, the ingredient in Benadryl, and that's what I recommend.

But my highest recommendation to people who find they no longer sleep like babies is to accept that adults don't sleep like babies. It's natural to sleep less efficiently as time goes on, and the wisest thing to do is to be flexible and learn to take naps in the daytime to make up for lost sleep at night. If you wake up and can't get back to sleep at night, read a book or listen to a tape.

I open the little bottle of Excedrin P.M. and notice a faint smell of vinegar. The tablets are changing color a bit, and one of them is crumbling. I notice now that the expiration date was eight years ago. The vinegar smell is no doubt from the aspirin breakdown in the Excedrin. I hate to think that people take tablets like this. In my opinion, old pills are not equivalent to stale food; they are equivalent to rotten food. Into the toilet they go.

Oh, oh! Another bottle of unfinished antibiotic, with my name on it. Here I am, a pharmacist, and I can't even follow the rules. The extremely important rule with antibiotics is to *finish the prescription!*

People get tired of taking pills, and as soon as they feel better, they tend to stop. They don't realize that the prescribed timing is carefully planned so that the infection will not just be stunted but actually destroyed. If you stop taking the antibiotic as soon as you feel better, the infection is apt to revive and be meaner and stronger than before. Then if your symptoms return and you finish your prescription, it's only enough to challenge the infection, not to knock it out. You have ruined the effectiveness of the cure by ignoring the proper timing.

Many people feel they should have some leftover antibiotic in the medicine cabinet just in case a need arises. That's not a good idea. Different antibiotics are needed to match different diagnoses. And things change so quickly in the field of antibiotics that your doctor may want to prescribe a new, improved one next time around.

Finally, here is a bottle of Ipecac Syrup I've never had to use, and I hope I'll never have to. But I wouldn't be without it until my children are all thoroughly trustworthy about what they are apt to taste and swallow. Poisoning is now the most common medical emergency among young children because of all the products around our homes.

I remember what happened to a friend several years ago. She walked into her bedroom one day and noticed immediately that her bottle of Tweed perfume was about three inches from where she kept it on top of a high chest of drawers. This struck her as peculiar, so she went over and checked it, but it looked untouched and nothing else was out of place.

Something urged her to go out into the yard and check her hyperactive two-year-old son, Jon, who was playing happily. She stuck her nose right up to his mouth and took a whiff. *Tweed!*

She ran in and called her pediatrician, who sent her to the drugstore for a bottle of Ipecac Syrup. She rushed home and forced the reluctant child to swallow a tablespoon of it, followed by a big glass of water. Then she took him back outside and started to play hard with him. He was rather pleased to have her urging him to run and run around the yard.

The doctor's directions worked perfectly, and after a few minutes of running, Jon stopped and got sick. His stomach was thoroughly emptied, and he was soon feeling fine again. The smell of Tweed vomit is uniquely pungent, and so Jon's mom gave away her bottle of Tweed to a friend and hopes never to smell that particular perfume again.

Because Ipecac Syrup isn't dependable if it is old, be sure to keep a fresh bottle on hand. First, check the product label of the swallowed substance to be certain that it is something that should be vomited before you use Ipecac. Then if your child is at least one-year-old, give him or her one tablespoon. Follow this dose with a lot of water, not milk, and then get the child to exercise until he or she vomits.

You should also keep the number of your poison control center by the telephone in case your child ever swallows something dangerous, since your physician or pharmacist might not be available to advise you. Remember that differing treatments are required for different kinds of poisons. Sometimes you don't want the child to vomit. (When in doubt as to what to do, take babies and young children to a hospital emergency room.)

And never assume that because you have a well-run household, your child won't eat or drink anything bizarre. Crazy things happen to even the most careful families. Any child is capable of doing something far-fetched sooner or later, such as swallowing medicine found in the trash. I imagine quite a long-running television program called "Can You Top This?" could be developed in which parents swap true stories of what their kids got into. Ipecac Syrup would be the perfect sponsor.

Worth Remembering

All things are poisons,
for there is nothing without poisonous qualities.
It is only the dose
which makes a thing a poison.
—Paraselsus[1]

BE PREPARED:
THE FIRST-AID KIT

In addition to having a well-stocked, current medicine cabinet, every family ought to have a first-aid kit to carry in the family car, or in a backpack while on a camping trip. It doesn't need to be large or fancy; it simply needs to be complete enough to meet basic first-aid needs. A kit that is five or six inches square should be sufficient for most families.

Here's my prescription for the essential items to be included in a good first-aid kit. One of the most helpful items is some kind of antibacterial ointment. You may be lucky enough to find this type of ointment in medicated strips so that you can pack your kit more compactly. These strips are especially handy since they only contain enough medication for one application on a normal scrape. It's usually difficult, however, to find these items unless you have a friendly doctor or pharmacist who is aware of your needs.

A tube of Neosporin (triple antibiotic ointment) or Polysporin (double antibiotic ointment) will do the trick. These products are safe to use on any kind of minor scrape, cut or burn.

If you're going on a camping trip, include some Foille burn ointment in your pack. You never know when you might burn your hand at the camp fire. Foille is also good for sunburn, though you may want to put in a bottle of Solarcaine lotion for that purpose. Pack these ointments only if they come in gels or plastic bottles. Aerosol spray cans in a first-aid kit are dangerous because they can explode.

I would also suggest you include rolls of half-inch and one-inch gauze. I recommend the stretchy-type gauze since it gives you more flexibility and is more adaptable for use in different situations. In addition, I would include a few two-by-two-inch, three-by-three-inch and four-by-four-inch gauze pads. The nonstick pads are best because they won't stick to an oozing wound.

These gauze pads usually come in bulk boxes. I would suggest you simply resupply your kit with these pads whenever you use one, rather than trying to pack fifty pads into your kit with all the other items you'll need.

Throw in half-inch and one-inch rolls of adhesive tape as well. Include a half-inch roll of paper tape, too. Paper tape is not as heavy as adhesive tape and is specially manufactured so as not to stick to a wound. With these varieties of tape types and sizes, you will have built-in flexibility to meet whatever need arises.

You'll also need a pair of surgical scissors to cut the gauze and bandages. It will be worth your while to invest in a good pair from your local pharmacy. Scissors that cut well ease stress during an emergency.

A single-edge razor blade can also be useful, particularly if it becomes necessary to cut off a piece of clothing to get better access to a wound. Try to find single-edge blades individually wrapped in protective cardboard or packaged in plastic dispensers. A pair of sharp, pointed, good quality tweezers should be tucked in along with your razor blade. A sterile needle is another excellent item to include.

For disinfecting purposes, your kit will need alcohol swabs; the kind used with diabetic syringes are about the right size. Besides the swabs, you'll want to carry a small bottle of cleansing solution, such as hydrogen peroxide or Hibiclens. This will allow you to clean and disinfect a wound if you are in a location where proper clean-up facilities are unavailable.

Include several sizes of bandages, too. You might simply wish to purchase one of those boxes of plastic strips that contains a variety of sizes and put a couple of each size in your pack. Be sure to include several knuckle bandages as well. Butterfly plastic bandages are excellent, too. If you sustain a cut deep enough to require stitches, butterfly strips can usually hold the cut together long enough for you to get medical assistance.

To be prepared for sprains, you'll want to include a couple of two-inch and four-inch Ace bandages. I recommend that you buy the self-adhesive kind or the ones with a Velcro strip. Otherwise, it's too easy to lose the clips that come with the regular Ace bandages.

Another useful item is a large triangular bandage. You can usually buy these prepackaged. Such a bandage can either be used as another Ace bandage or as a nice sling in the event you break your arm.

For the inevitable problem of blisters, I recommend a product called Spenco blister kit, which treats the problem by operating as a sort of second skin. (You can find these kits at your local sporting goods store.) It works nicely and comes packaged flat so that it fits easily into a compact space.

In addition, you'll want to include an instant cold pack. They are excellent for sprains or any other type of injury that requires cold therapy. Cold packs keep forever until you use them. If you need them, you simply crush the contents and mix, and you have a cold pack that remains very cold for an hour or two.

For pain relievers, I recommend small bottles of aspirin, acetaminophen and ibuprofen products. I think aspirin is the best thing you can use for a headache. If you have young children, however, you'll want to use Children's Tylenol Chewable Tablets because they are easier to tolerate.

Ibuprofen products are excellent for a toothache, but they're particularly useful if you sprain your ankle because they help to reduce the inflammation and local swelling. Ibuprofen offers the added benefit of relieving menstrual cramps.

Besides pain medication, I would pack a small supply of antacid tablets and cold tablets to take care of some of the discomforts that often occur on a camping trip.

A couple of small packets of smelling salts are also useful additions to the family first-aid kit. You can usually buy small packets that you simply crush whenever you are faced with the need.

You may also want to include a thermometer in your kit. The forehead temperature strips might work, but they tend not to be very accurate. It's just as easy to use a regular thermometer, which wouldn't take up much room. Buy a thermometer that comes with a plastic case to help protect against breakage. (Be sure to disinfect your thermometer with alcohol swabs after using it.)

Another item that could come in handy is an eye wash. It's not unusual for something to get in someone's eye during an outing. An application of an eye wash could quickly alleviate that problem. I recommend Collyrium for Fresh Eyes because it comes with an eye cup for convenience, and it's an excellent product.

If you plan to hike, include a tube or individual strips of 0.5 percent hydrocortisone cream to treat insect bites or poison oak rash. Hydrocortisone works wonders on all sorts of rashes, hives or skin reactions. Cortaid or CaldeCORT Anti-Itch Cream are two good products that relieve itching related to the above conditions.

Nowadays, I think it's also wise to include some kind of chemical wash, in the event you inadvertently encounter some toxic chemicals. This wash is useful for your eyes or your skin.

A small sewing kit for repair jobs, a few safety pins and several cotton-tipped swabs are good to include. Such items leave you well prepared for almost any emergency.

Several excellent ready-made first-aid kits are available. A kit as comprehensive as the one I have suggested, however, would probably be expensive. If you prepare your own, you can save considerably.

After you have purchased or created your kit, update it periodically. Be sure to watch the expiration dates on the medication you include. I also suggest that you check your kit every time you go on a trip. It might even be helpful to develop your own checklist as to what should be included so that you don't inadvertently overlook an important item. Taking just a few minutes to do this could end up saving your life.

I remember one Sunday at a church picnic, my son fell on a rock while playing with his friends. He sustained a nasty gash in his forehead. Blood was running everywhere, and we knew we needed to stop it as quickly as possible. Someone ran for the church's first-aid kit. Unfortunately, it was in a complete shambles. It hadn't been restocked in years, and Band-Aid wrappers lay everywhere. We couldn't possibly have found what we needed amidst all the clutter and empty boxes. Luckily, Dad was able to come to the rescue, but it taught me a good lesson about keeping one's first-aid kit stocked.

FIRST-AID KIT CONTENTS

Small Kit	Moderate Kit	Ultra-Deluxe Kit
1. Antibacterial ointment: Neosporin Mycitracin Polysporin	1. Antibacterial ointment: Neosporin Mycitracin Polysporin	1. Antibacterial ointment: Neosporin Mycitracin Polysporin
2. 1/2", 1" gauze rolls (flexible)	2. 1/2", 1" gauze rolls (flexible)	2. 1/2", 1" gauze rolls (flexible)
3. 2" gauze pads	3. 2" gauze pads, 4" gauze pads	3. 2" gauze pads, 4" gauze pads
4. Alcohol swabs or first-aid cleansing swabs	4. Alcohol swabs or first-aid cleansing swabs	4. Alcohol swabs or first-aid cleansing swabs
5. Bandages—1" plastic strips and junior strips	5. Bandages—1" plastic strips and junior strips	5. Bandages—1" plastic strips and junior strips
6. Small plastic bottle of hydrogen peroxide	6. Small plastic bottle of hydrogen peroxide	6. Small plastic bottle of hydrogen peroxide
7. Scissors	7. Scissors, razor blade	7. Scissors, razor blade
8. 1/2" roll adhesive tape	8. Adhesive tape: 1/2", 1" roll; paper tape: 1/2"	8. Adhesive tape: 1/2", 1" roll; paper tape: 1/2"
	9. Burn ointment: Foille	9. Burn ointment: Foille
	10. Ace-type, self-adhesive bandages: 2", 4"	10. Ace-type, self-adhesive bandages: 2", 4"
	11. Instant cold pack	11. Instant cold pack
	12. Aspirin, Tylenol	12. Aspirin, Tylenol
	13. Smelling salts	13. Smelling salts
	14. Sterile needle	14. Sterile needle
	15. Bandages, including knuckle, strips, spots, etc.	15. Bandages, including knuckle, strips, spots, etc.

Small Kit	Moderate Kit	Ultra-Deluxe Kit
	16. Butterfly and triangular bandages	16. Butterfly and triangular bandages
	17. Thermometer	17. Thermometer
	18. Eye wash: Collyrium for Fresh Eyes	18. Eye wash: Collyrium for Fresh Eyes
	19. Tweezers	19. Tweezers
	20. Hydrocortisone cream 0.5%: Cortaid, CaldeCORT Anti-Itch Cream	20. Hydrocortisone cream 0.5%: Cortaid, CaldeCORT Anti-Itch Cream
	21. Spenco blister kit	21. Spenco blister kit
		22. Chemical wash
		23. Cold tablets
		24. Eye pads
		25. Small sewing kit
		26. Antacid tablets

Worth Remembering

He heals the brokenhearted,
and binds up their wounds.
—*Psalms 147:3, RSV*

QUESTIONS
AND ANSWERS

I find myself answering patrons' questions from A to Z all year long. The following questions represent examples of ones I hear in the drugstore. Most of them came to me in the mail after I was interviewed by Dr. James Dobson on the Focus on the Family radio broadcast.

Dear Dan Little,

I am pregnant, and I don't know which medicines are safe to take. My allergies have me congested, with a stuffy nose, sore throat and a cough that racks my body. I called the pharmacist at my local discount store, and he told me to take cough syrup and a decongestant like Sudafed.

So I did that, and for three nights I was dizzy, unable to sleep, painful in all my joints and scared. I felt that if I didn't think about breathing, I would accidentally stop.

It was terrible, because I couldn't sleep at night in that condition, and in the daytime I had my three-year-old to take care of. Finally I stopped all the medication, and that night I slept like a baby, even with all my allergy symptoms back.

My question is, what should I take for my allergies? Also, what other kinds of medicines are safe to take for pain or sleep problems when I am pregnant? Thank you so very much.

Sincerely Yours,

Mrs. Sally Cook

Dear Mrs. Cook,

Your question is a wise one. I assume that you are too young to remember the thalidomide tragedy of the 1960s. Thousands of babies were born deformed because of a "safe" medication that doctors prescribed to healthy pregnant women. Diethylstilbestrol (DES) was another "safe" medication for pregnant women, and it ended up causing uterine cancer in the next generation.

Your question reminds me of a true story from my early years as a pharmacist. I was working in a local chain store with a slender technician who became pregnant. She planned to work through her pregnancy, but she developed severe morning sickness. She started out with the standard morning-sickness medication at that time, but she became so nauseated she couldn't stay in the pharmacy. Her doctors then switched her to a strong emetic that is not to be used by pregnant women unless under a doctor's supervision. Instead of getting better, she got worse. She not only could not come to work, but she also could not get out of bed.

She ended up in the hospital with severe dehydration, IV's and every possible medication to try to control the nausea and severe vomiting. After a few weeks things calmed down, and she went home.

One day she came into the pharmacy while I was at work. She

looked like a frail, thin, stick of a girl, with a faint smile on her face. She was glad to be alive.

Several months later, after a long battle, she gave birth to a healthy baby with no apparent problems. I shudder to think of all the medication that pregnant mother had taken, but of course her life had been in jeopardy so there was no choice.

I may sound harsh, but my answer to pregnant women with allergy, pain, nausea or sleep problems is one word: "Suffer." Don't take any medication unless it's absolutely necessary for your health. This is especially important during the first three months, but during the whole pregnancy you must be careful.

Believe it or not, even aspirin can be detrimental to the baby's respiratory system during the last trimester.

When my wife was pregnant with our second child, she took Bendectin for one week to relieve morning sickness and then stopped. She also took one Tylenol and that was it. She had severe water retention, but her physicians said no diuretics.

Because we wanted our children to be exposed to as little medication as possible, we were very careful. My wife is a coffee drinker, but she gave up coffee throughout her three pregnancies. Caffeine has been shown to cause birth defects in animals and seems to increase premature deliveries and low birth weights. Of course, smoking during pregnancy is risky to the baby in several ways. I say no coffee, tea, caffeinated-colas, alcohol, cigarettes or medicine for the average pregnant woman. *Nothing is without potential side effects.*

I warn especially against tetracycline. It can harm the mother's liver and can also cause discolored and mottled teeth in the child and defective bone development.

Of course, certain women need to take medicine during pregnany—for preexisting medical conditions or infections that come along during pregnancy, for example. Toxemia is extremely dangerous and must be treated.

In conclusion, my advice for pregnant women is to check with their physicians and take as little medication as possible. No effort should be spared to protect the mother's life, but the welfare of the unborn child should come ahead of the mother's comfort. Good luck with your pregnancy and your growing family!

Dear Mr. Little,

I wondered if you could answer a question that has been troubling me for a few months. I had pushed it to the back of my mind, but it surfaced after hearing you on the radio and reading an article that spoke of the dangers of overuse of antibiotics.

When we took my son for his first appointment with a dermatologist in December, he prescribed tetracycline for our son's acne, two capsules a day the first month, and one a day since then. I expressed my concern, but the doctor just brushed me off as if I were an overanxious mother to doubt or ask questions.

Do you think it could be harmful to our son to keep taking that indefinitely? My husband, who had severe acne as a teenager, has been taking tetracycline for years and has stomach problems.

Our son has been so healthy these last couple of years—I don't want anything to hurt his immune system or his stomach.

Cordially,
Jan Stein

Dear Mrs. Stein,

I get concerned about the preoccupation with teenage acne. (I'm not talking about the severe types of acne that can scar.) Teenagers and their parents spend hundreds of dollars on prescriptions that will be taken for months and maybe years, for a problem that looks pretty minor to me.

My personal prejudice is definitely not to use antibiotics unless absolutely necessary. According to the University of Southern California drug information center, some long-term effects on the immune system can occur with consistent use of some antibiotics for acne. Documented studies, however, have not been done.

In severe cases of acne, the medication Accutane, a prescription drug and a powerful cousin of vitamin A, is very effective. The trouble with Accutane is that it has severe side effects and is very expensive. It should be used only for recalcitrant cystic acne, and its use should be closely monitored by a physician. I'm glad to say that Accutane has proved to be a wonderful answer for many of the most extreme cases of acne. But it should *never* be used by a woman who might become pregnant, as severe birth defects are almost certain to occur.

Dear Mr. Little,

Last week, I heard you on the radio while I was driving to an appointment. You gave some very practical advice. I thought you could tell me how to solve an embarrassing problem I can't seem to correct. I'm a salesman, and when I meet clients I need to look my best, but I have a severe case of dandruff.

I have been using a shampoo with coal tar in it, however, you warned that it can cause premature balding. You recommended Zincon shampoo, but I couldn't find it in my local supermarket. Please advise me where I can purchase it or any other good dandruff shampoos. I'd appreciate all the information you can give to help me with this problem.

Respectfully,
Tom Hudson

Dear Mr. Hudson:

A good coal-tar shampoo may indeed be the product of choice for severe itchy, scaly scalp conditions once you have been examined by a physician. Denorex, Zetar and Ionil-T are all good tar-based shampoos.

When your dandruff is under control, or if you would like a moderate medicated shampoo, Zincon is an excellent choice. Zincon is manufactured by the Lederle Laboratories, and I have used it for years. You should be able to find all these products at your local pharmacy, or ask the pharmacist to order them for you.

Dear Dan Little,

Yesterday, I heard you before I went to school. Could you help me? I have acne. I tried the special soaps, but they dried my skin out and made it look worse. Now I use Clearasil cleanser, which works better. Do you know about any other cleansers that aren't too harsh? What else can I do to get rid of this acne? Boys don't like girls who have it, so I'd really like to know what to do real soon.

Thanks,
Christy Anderson

Dear Miss Anderson:

Acne soaps and acne preparations tend to dry out the skin. That is part of their purpose. When dryness becomes a problem, some excellent cleansers help fight it. These include: Purpose Soap, Oilatum Soap and Lowila Cake. Along with your doctor's care and eating healthy foods, these products should help you.

Dear Mr. Little:

During the Focus on the Family radio program, you suggested that people avoid deodorants with aluminum. I looked at the anti-

*perspirant I use and saw that the number one ingredient is
aluminum. I went to the drugstore and looked at the deodorants
on the shelf, but they had it, too. What would you use?*

Thanks for sharing so much helpful information.

Sincerely,

Mrs. Donna Townsend

Dear Mrs. Townsend,

Aluminum was by far the most popular topic of inquiry in both
calls and letters after my radio talks. It's true that Alzheimer's
patients are reported to have high aluminum concentrations in their
brains. This is just an observation; it doesn't prove any link
between aluminum in our deodorants and Alzheimer's disease.

But I would suggest not cooking in aluminum pans and not using
a lot of antacids, to cut down aluminum intake. (If a doctor tells
a patient to take antacids regularly for a physical problem, that's
another matter.) I've chosen to use a simple deodorant instead of
an antiperspirant, because I can't find any aluminum-free anti-
perspirants. I don't have a problem with wetness under my arms.
If I did, I would probably alternate between plain deodorant and
an antiperspirant.

Dear Mr. Little,

*A while ago, I had a bad sinus infection. The doctor put me on
amoxicillin, and it worked so well I felt better in a few hours. A
week later, however, when I was about done with the pills, I broke
out with a rash all over my body. I took Benadryl for the reaction,
which worked fine. The doctor told me I was allergic to amoxicillin
and that I shouldn't take it again.*

*Recently, I had another sore throat and tonsillitis. This time I
saw a different doctor, and he said that since I was allergic to*

amoxicillin, he didn't want to take any chances with penicillin. Does this mean I'm allergic to penicillin, too? When I had the reaction before, the doctor said that it was caused by the "bonding" material in the amoxicillin. Are there any other penicillin-based medications I could take when I need an antibiotic? The amoxicillin worked so well, and the alternative medications are so expensive.
   Sincerely,
   Donald Brown

Dear Mr. Brown,
   There's more to your question than meets the eye. Indeed, the most common allergic reaction to penicillin is a red, itchy rash. But amoxicillin and some other antibiotics have their own rash as a side effect that is not an allergic reaction. It's very difficult to tell the difference.
   A patient calls and tells the physician that a red rash has developed. The physician says to stop the medication, and in two days the rash is gone. But was it actually an allergic reaction? Who knows!
   Many patients who are not allergic to the medications still have reactions such as pain or nausea. Unfortunately, these people never use the medications again because of a nonexistent allergy. Always remember that some side effects are not really allergic reactions after all.

Dear Dan Little,
   Can you tell us if an over-the-counter medication exists to help the sneezing and runny nose of hay fever but has something other than antihistamine in it?
   My husband has no serious allergy problem, just days when he

sneezes and his nose runs constantly. He is a mail carrier (in a truck), and he feels miserable in this condition.

All the over-the-counter drugs so far have knocked him out. Our best luck was with Alka-Seltzer Plus Cold Medicine, which gave him relief and mild sleepiness. But the warning on it about prostate problems makes us afraid to continue with it.

Going to an allergist is such a long, drawn-out process that it doesn't seem worth the effort for his problem. I have asthma, and getting diagnosed and treated for it through a local hospital seemed to take forever.

Isn't there some over-the-counter medication that can ease his symptoms without making him a zombie or endangering his prostate?
Cordially,
Lisa Franklin

Dear Mrs. Franklin,

Runny nose, sneezing and watery eyes are caused by allergens (pollen, dust, cat hair and such). Allergens cause the mast cells in the body to break down and release histamine, which gives patients mild to severe reactions. This is where we get the word antihistamine. These medications try to neutralize the body's histamine reaction. Unfortunately, antihistamines can cause considerable drowsiness or light-headedness.

First, I suggest that your husband try lowering his dose. Cut the tablet in half or open the capsule and pour out part of the powder.

Second, I suggest Dimetane tablets, which seem to have slightly milder side effects than most other antihistamines.

Third, a new prescription medication called Seldane may help. It seems to be quite a breakthrough. Many patients are finally able to get allergy relief without the side effects from older antihistamine products. Seldane does, however, have two drawbacks. It's expensive, and people vary so much that some patients will still have side effects. But in my opinion, Seldane is far and away the best product on the market today.

Regarding the warning about prostate problems on the Alka-Seltzer Plus label, the decongestant in this product can cause enlargement of the prostate gland. This will cause increased urinary retention, which can lead to serious problems. The medicine doesn't affect the prostate gland. But it will aggravate the prostate even more, if it was already enlarged due to a preexisting condition.

Dear Mr. Little,

I hope that you can settle some confusion for me. I am a tennis player, and it gets mighty hot in the summer here. My dad was active in sports when he was young, and he urges me to take salt tablets during summer sports activities as his coaches told him to do. He said salted popcorn or peanuts are a good idea on hot days also. It's to replace all the salt we lose when we perspire, so we won't get weak.

My tennis coach is young, and he said it's not a good idea to use all that salt. I don't want to argue with either one of them. But I do want to do what is really best. Do you have any advice?

Also, one of my friends got an infected blister and had to miss some games. What do you suggest in case I get a blister?

Yours,
Jerry Norman

Dear Mr. Norman,

I wish I could take back all the wrong advice I gave on this topic in the past. I grew up with the teaching that salt tablets are good for active people in hot weather. My brother used to take salt tablets when he played high school football. I advised people to take them.

Then recently I went to a sports medicine seminar and listened to a sports nutritionist who had been in the Olympic marathon trials herself. She told us that the usefulness of salt tablets in sweaty sports is a myth. All this salt in the stomach tends to pull water out of your system into your stomach, which makes your dehydration worse. Instead of taking salt, you should just drink water.

Your friend should have kept his blister clean and dry and loosely covered if possible. Some products out now also help. I particularly recommend the blister kit from Spenco. Look for it in your pharmacy or in an athletic store. I recommend that you get one and keep it on hand for yourself.

Dear Dan Little,

After all these years, I just saw on the label of a bottle of antibiotic that it should be refrigerated. Is that an important rule that we weren't warned about before? Should other medications be refrigerated also?

Thank you,
Sarah Springer

Dear Mrs. Springer,

No, don't refrigerate all medications! In fact, only certain antibiotics should be refrigerated, and others should *not*. Always read the directions carefully, and ask your pharmacist about proper storage temperatures for your specific medicines if the label doesn't tell you.

Worth Remembering

The only stupid question is the one that was not asked.
—Anonymous

CHRONIC ILLNESSES: FINDING THE BALM IN GILEAD

Every workday, I am aware of the endless stories of human lives that touch my counter. That's why I like to do more than just hand the patient a bag and take the money. Each person is a fascinating story, each person is a parable I can learn from, and each person is someone I can help, even though sometimes only in limited ways.

Some of the people I've encountered have chronic illnesses. For them, a trip to the medicine cabinet or to the drugstore will not solve their problem. I'd like you to meet some of the individuals who have learned to deal with issues of health from a perspective most of us hope we'll never have to. But the truth is, most of us will, at some point in our lives, find ourselves with an incurable ailment.

Nancy Washburn was one of the most vivacious, friendly customers I had in the six and a half years I ran my drugstore. When I found out, during one of our discussions, that she had a glass eye, I asked her for more details about her medical history.

This courageous, twenty-four-year-old lady, who had given herself the nickname "Popeye," was an instruction book for anyone battling a chronic disease or disability, showing how to live productively, positively and with dignity.

Nancy's story began in the summer of her tenth year. She was scrawny but active, with outstanding health. That summer she developed a voracious appetite, but she kept losing weight. She began drinking a lot of water and urinating more frequently.

Then one night on a family camping trip, Nancy got up to urinate and filled an entire coffee can that her parents had left in the tent. At the age of ten, weighing only forty-five pounds, Nancy was diagnosed as having diabetes.

Within a couple of days, Nancy started taking insulin. She didn't mind. After all, she was the first kid on the block to give herself a shot.

I advise parents of diabetic children like Nancy to help them learn about their disease and to make sure they participate in their own care. Children will make mistakes, but they need to understand the relationship between care and the disease's complications.

More reliable tests exist today than in Nancy's first years, so it's easier to know what one's blood-sugar count is. While the testing kits are expensive, some insurance companies will pay for them. Blood results are immediate, and some patients check up to six times a day to find out when the blood sugar spikes or plummets.

Also because diabetics have to watch what they eat all the time, the disease can lead to bulimia or anorexia. A person doesn't lose a taste for sugar when he or she becomes a diabetic, and sometimes eating disorders develop as a person attempts to avoid "bad" foods by not eating anything or by vomiting after eating them.

In 1979 Nancy began laser treatment for her eyes. She was having leakage and bleeding, because diabetes causes the blood vessels in the eyes to deteriorate. For 80 percent of diabetics, laser treatment can prevent blindness. But Nancy was in the 20 percent.

Rather than isolating herself from others, she went for bus rides, traveling from thirty to a hundred miles a day. Her senses became more real this way, and she developed her independence. She also started walking five to ten miles a day to better control her diabetes.

Nancy visited an ocularist, an artist who makes and fits artificial eyes. Unfortunately, she developed a painful staph infection that became so severe that it could have perforated her retina or infected her brain. For two months her parents drove her to the doctor's office every day for two shots in her eye. The blindness, pain and helplessness made this the worst period in Nancy's life. She had no strength left and had to grab on to other people for faith and prayer.

Eventually Nancy began to recover and went to a new ocularist. While she was recuperating and going to the doctor, she suddenly started to see things whizzing by in her peripheral vision. She was startled and excited all at once.

Little by little, she could see more. In a year, her vision went from 20/200 to 20/60 and then, with glasses, to 20/40. That's exactly what she needed to drive her car again. So not only was one of her greatest longings fulfilled—to see people's expressions again—but she also got to read and drive herself places.

Unfortunately, she also suffered from neuropathies (in which the nerves become diseased). Her extremities were numb and painful because the nerve signals were altered.

In 1987 she walked barefoot out to a swimming pool. Because her feet were numb, she didn't feel the heat of the pavement, and because of her diabetes, her skin burned easily. She suffered third-degree burns on her feet.

During her long recuperation she gained weight again, lost strength and suffered hip calcification. That left her weaker than ever. But Nancy fought back and, with much hard work, rose above her complications. At this point in life she would like to reactivate her RN license and represent an insulin pump company.

As Nancy says, there is no rest from diabetes—no rest for the person who has it, and no rest for family members. But Popeye always smiles, always laughs, always has something funny to say. She is an example to many others, a wonderful lady with great dignity.

Two other patients besides Popeye have especially inspired me as I've watched them handle crushing misfortune—Barbara Uditsky and Pann Baltz.

Barbara is a middle-aged woman with muscular dystrophy. I had owned my store a year or so when she first came in. I couldn't quite see the doorway, but I heard the door open and then heard a metal clanking sound coming down the aisle.

I looked over the counter and saw a woman about five-foot-one. She was using arm crutches and braces to walk. She had fought her disease for years. At one time she had gone for counseling, and a neurologist and psychologist told her to stand up and yell at the top of her lungs. She did it and released five years of nonacceptance of her disease. The experience was a breakthrough for her.

She could barely walk and had heart trouble, but she was able to drive her car, do some light bookkeeping, and—best of all—play the piano at her church. She absolutely loved to play the piano; it was her source of joy.

As years passed, Barbara kept me up on her setbacks and surgeries and the decline in the use of her hands and legs. She had to take medicine for depression and heart trouble. When she could no longer play the piano at her church, she felt terrible. But she smiled a wonderful smile at me and said, "I know the Lord's working. It's okay; He's giving me the strength."

Barbara eventually lost everything that most of us value in life—the ability to walk, drive and earn money. But she knows that the Lord is in control, and she loves Him dearly. Her life is an example of how to live through tragedy and despair.

Pann Baltz, a vibrant elementary school teacher in her thirties, had an uncanny string of calamities in her life. Because her legs are partly paralyzed from a heart condition, she walks with braces and crutches. She has had many surgeries and has almost lost her life. As if that weren't enough, when she was stopped for a traffic light, a utility truck ran into her and badly damaged her back and foot.

Then she had a freak accident with a piece of See's candy. When she bit into it, one whole side of her jaw fractured into several pieces. She had to go through a bone implant and reconstruction of her jaw, and when the procedure didn't work, she had to have her jaw rebroken and go through it again.

Pann's mother used to come down from Seattle to take care of her in some of these traumatic times, and she has stood at my counter with tears running down her cheeks, wondering how much more Pann would have to go through. We all wondered. They say that lightning really does strike twice (or more) in the same place sometimes. Pann is one of those people who keeps getting hit.

Her latest calamity was a blood disorder similar to leukemia. She was trying to get it under control with chemotherapy. When the doctors were injecting a caustic kind of chemotherapy into her arm, something went wrong and the chemical severely damaged the skin and tissues of her hand.

The last time I saw her, her hand and arm were shaking with pain, and you could see the strain in her face. Yet through all her calamities, she was a dominant force for living, and she said, "This isn't going to stop me." She was still full of life, still eager to share all she had with her elementary school students.

My collection of pharmacy medicines is totally inadequate to cope with the needs of people like Popeye, Barbara and Pann, who get hit by such physical misfortunes. I stand in awe of their courage and faith in God. These three are to me an example of how Christ would handle physical adversity.

People like Popeye, Barbara and Pann inspire me and turn my work as a pharmacist into a ministry. As I have been working on this book, I have found myself reflecting often on my father's life. He has been dead almost three years now, but the legacy he left behind is an ever-present reality.

The other day I happened across his diary. I had read these pages before, but somehow I felt different this time. I was deeply moved as I read of his decision to become a relief missionary doctor in Swaziland.

One weekend he attended a Los Angeles District laymen's retreat for the Nazarene church where he heard a doctor recount his experience as a medical missionary to Swaziland. For some reason, this doctor's presentation really gripped my dad's heart. He couldn't shake the feeling that God wanted to send him to Swaziland, also. He gave God every excuse in the book as to why this was not a feasible plan.

But every excuse he stated reminded him of an earlier promise he had given to God that he would do anything God needed him to do. So in February 1962, my dad followed through on his promise to God.

My father took off from Los Angeles International Airport by himself for six weeks in Africa. When he left, he had no idea how he was going to get from Johannesburg, South Africa, to

Swaziland, but he was met by some missionaries at the Johannesburg airport who took him straight to Swaziland.

Those next six weeks changed his life. He was exposed to all sorts of medical problems he had never encountered in America. But what most profoundly affected him was the sacrifice of the missionaries and their ability to be resourceful. His diary is filled with accounts of his admiration for the medical staff.

When my father returned to America, he was forced to face another crisis. My seventeen-year-old brother, who unknowingly was suffering from a congenital heart abnormality, died while swimming in our pool. To lose his precious son so suddenly and at such a tender age was almost more than my father could handle, but the memory of his missionary friends in Swaziland struggling against all odds sustained him in his darkest hours.

In loving memory of my brother, my father established a fund to finance some of the needs of these medical missionaries in Swaziland. As a result, the missionaries were able to purchase land to upgrade and expand the clinic.

As I think of my father boarding that plane for Africa without having any idea how he was going to get to his final destination, I am reminded of Peter and his water-walking experience. This incident in Peter's life has often been used as an example of lack of faith. But it seems to me, as I reread the story, that Peter's actions represent a great deal of faith. It took a lot of courage to get out of the boat. Peter's major mistake was that once he was on the water, he was so impressed by his water-walking skills that he forgot to focus his attention on Jesus.

I am beginning to understand that God is calling me to get out of my boat, to not be satisfied with the normal everyday transactions of a local pharmacy, but to look beyond to the greater needs in the world. I believe he is calling me to pick up where my father left off in Swaziland. I am not a doctor, so I can't give in the same way he did. But as a pharmacist, I can help supply medications and medical supplies that the missionaries so desperately need.

I always liked the old black spiritual "There Is a Balm in Gilead." It is the perfect hymn for pharmacists and patients.

> Sometimes I feel discouraged
> And think my work's in vain,
> But then the Holy Spirit
> Revives my soul again.
> There is a balm in Gilead
> To make the wounded whole;
> There is a balm in Gilead
> To heal the sin-sick soul.
> If you can't preach like Peter,
> If you can't pray like Paul,
> Just tell the love of Jesus,
> And say He died for all.
> There is a balm in Gilead
> To make the wounded whole;
> There is a balm in Gilead
> To heal the sin-sick soul.
> —*Traditional spiritual*

God is in the healing business both physically and spiritually and will be until everyone is perfectly healed forever. The song "There is a Balm in Gilead" claims that Jesus and His love for us are the medicine that really heals. Medicine for the soul.

One of the most important gifts we can give one another is to stand with those who are lonely or sick, offering them words of cheer and reassurance. That's one of the best medicines a pharmacist or anyone else has to offer.

We all have the prescription: "Love one another."

<u>Worth Remembering</u>

A friend loves at all times.
—*Proverbs 17:17a, NIV*

NOTES

Chapter 1
1. Max A. Fern and Betty Fern, *How to Save Dollars with Generic Drugs* (New York: William Morrow and Company, 1985) 237.
2. Barbara B. Huff et al., eds., *PDR Edition 1989: Physicians' Desk Reference for Non-Prescription Drugs* (Ordall: Medical Economics Company Inc., 1989) 651, 691.
3. Ibid.
4. Mark Twain, *The Complete Humorous Sketches and Tales of Mark Twain,* Edited by Charles Neider (Garden City: Doubleday & Co., Inc., 1961) 25-26.
5. M. Laurence Lieberman, *The Essential Guide to Generic Drugs* (New York: Harper & Row Publishers, Inc., 1986) 2.

Chapter 2
1. John Bartlett, *Familiar Quotations,* Edited by Emily Morison Beck (Boston: Little, Brown and Company, 1968) 324.

Chapter 3
1. James W. Long, M.D., *The Essential Guide to Prescription Drugs: 1989* (New York: Harper & Row Publishers, Inc., 1989) 610-613.
2. Bartlett, *Familiar Quotations,* 1017.

Chapter 6
1. Marlene Soronsky, *Season's Greetings* (New York: Harper & Row Publishers, Inc. 1986) 81.

Chapter 7
1. Bartlett, *Familiar Quotations,* 326.

Chapter 8
1. Paul E. Schindler, Jr., *Aspirin Therapy: Cutting the Risk of Heart Disease* (New York: Walker and Company, 1978) 33-42.
2. Helen Klusek Hamilton, et al., eds., *Professional Guide to Diseases* (Springhouse: Intermed Communications Inc., 1982) 624.
3. Bartlett, *Familiar Quotations,* 817.

Chapter 9
1. Bartlett, *Familiar Quotations,* 187.

Chapter 10
1. Fern and Fern, *How to Save Dollars,* 16.

2 . Lieberman, *Essential Guide*, 11.

3 . Paul Tournier, *The Healing of Persons* (New York: Harper & Row Publishers, Inc., 1965) 218.

Chapter 11

1 . George Seldes, compiler *The Great Quotations* (New York: Pocket Books, 1972) 733.

INDEX